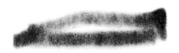

The Johns Hopkins
Breast Cancer Handbook

for Health Care Professionals

Lillie D. Shockney, RN, BS, MAS

Administrative Director
The Johns Hopkins Avon Foundation Comprehensive Breast Center
Baltimore, MD

Theodore N. Tsangaris, MD

Associate Professor of Surgery
Chief of Breast Surgery
Director, The Johns Hopkins Avon Foundation Comprehensive Breast Center
Baltimore, MD

JONES AND BARTLETT PUBLISHERS

Sudbury, Massachusetts

BOSTON   TORONTO   LONDON   SINGAPORE

World Headquarters

Jones and Bartlett Publishers	Jones and Bartlett Publishers	Jones and Bartlett Publishers
40 Tall Pine Drive	Canada	International
Sudbury, MA 01776	6339 Ormindale Way	Barb House, Barb Mews
978-443-5000	Mississauga, Ontario L5V 1J2	London W6 7PA
info@jbpub.com	Canada	United Kingdom
www.jbpub.com		
United Kingdom		

Jones and Bartlett's books and products are available through most bookstores and online booksellers. To contact Jones and Bartlett Publishers directly, call 800-832-0034, fax 978-443-8000, or visit our website www.jbpub.com.

Substantial discounts on bulk quantities of Jones and Bartlett's publications are available to corporations, professional associations, and other qualified organizations. For details and specific discount information, contact the special sales department at Jones and Bartlett via the above contact information or send an email to specialsales@jbpub.com.

The authors, editor, and publisher have made every effort to provide accurate information. However, they are not responsible for errors, omissions, or for any outcomes related to the use of the contents of this book and take no responsibility for the use of the products and procedures described. Treatments and side effects described in this book may not be applicable to all people; likewise, some people may require a dose or experience a side effect that is not described herein. Drugs and medical devices are discussed that may have limited availability controlled by the Food and Drug Administration (FDA) for use only in a research study or clinical trial. Research, clinical practice, and government regulations often change the accepted standard in this field. When consideration is being given to use of any drug in the clinical setting, the health care provider or reader is responsible for determining FDA status of the drug, reading the package insert, and reviewing prescribing information for the most up-to-date recommendations on dose, precautions, and contraindications, and determining the appropriate usage for the product. This is especially important in the case of drugs that are new or seldom used.

Production Credits

Executive Publisher: Christopher Davis
Production Director: Amy Rose
Associate Editor: Kathy Richardson
Production Editor: Diana Coe
Associate Marketing Manager: Rebecca Wasley
Editorial Assistant: Jessica Acox
Manufacturing Buyer: Therese Connell
Cover Design: Kate Ternullo
Cover Image: © Photos.com
Composition: ATLIS Graphics
Printing and Binding: Malloy, Inc.
Cover Printing: Malloy, Inc.

Library of Congress Cataloging-in-Publication Data
Shockney, Lillie, 1953-
    The Johns Hopkins breast cancer handbook for health care professionals / Lillie D. Shockney and Theodore N. Tsangaris. — 1st ed.
        p. ; cm.
    Includes bibliographical references and index.
    ISBN-13: 978-0-7637-4992-7
    ISBN-10: 0-7637-4992-3
    1. Breast-Cancer-Handbooks, manuals, etc.   I. Tsangaris, Theodore N.   II. Title.
III. Title: Breast cancer handbook for health care professionals.
    [DNLM: 1. Breast Neoplasms-therapy. 2. Breast Neoplasms. WP 870 S559j 2008]
    RC280.B8S49515 2008
    616.99′449—dc22   2007040638

6048

Printed in the United States of America
11 10 09 08 07   10 9 8 7 6 5 4 3 2 1

Dedication

I consider it a privilege to care for breast cancer patients during the most vulnerable time in their lives and so I dedicate this book to all of the primary care doctors, nurses, gynecologists, and other clinicians who will be sharing the responsibility of caring for these patients as they continue their medical journey as long-term breast cancer survivors.

I also wish to thank all of the contributing authors for the great deal of time and effort given to share their expertise. As a united team we can collectively help ensure that breast cancer survivors will feel confident about their ongoing care.

Lillie D. Shockney, RN, BS, MAS

Contents

CHAPTER **1**

Selecting a Breast Center to Refer Patients
Lillie D. Shockney, RN, BS, MAS

CHAPTER **2**

Diagnostic Evaluation/Image Guided Biopsies
Nagi F. Khouri, MD

CHAPTER **3**

Understanding Breast Pathology
Pedram Argani, MD

CHAPTER **4**

Breast Cancer: Surgical Options and Management
Theodore N. Tsangaris, MD

Preface

Breast cancer remains the most common malignancy and one of the most feared diseases in American women. Thanks to advances in screening and therapy, the mortality rate from breast cancer is dropping, and it appears that age-adjusted incidence is also decreasing. Estimates for 2007 from the American Cancer Society (ACS) suggest that approximately 180,000 women will be diagnosed with invasive breast cancer and an estimated 44,000 women will receive a diagnosis of in situ cancer, largely ductal carcinoma in situ (DCIS). Approximately 40,000 women will succumb to the disease but most survive. Indeed, in 2002, breast cancer survivors accounted for only 22% of the approximately 10 million cancer survivors with invasive cancers. These statistics imply that many primary care, gynecology, and internal medicine physicians and advanced practitioners will be involved in the assessment, diagnosis, treatment, and long-term evaluation of such patients.

Breast cancer diagnosis and treatment is a rapidly evolving field. This book is designed to provide succinct information about breast health assessment, when and how to refer a patient in need of diagnostic breast evaluation, types of therapy that patients may receive, how treatment might affect other medical conditions, and the role of surveillance during and after treatment. It also contains specialized topics such as menopausal management, examination of reconstructed or radiated breasts, and evidence-based follow-up algorithms. Primary care physicians, gynecologists, and other health care professionals play an important role in the care and monitoring of breast cancer survivors after treatment is completed, because they are in a position to address the full spectrum of the cancer survivor's health needs. In fact, randomized trials conducted in the United

Kingdom and Canada show that survival for patients who have completed initial management for early breast cancer is equal whether they are followed by their cancer specialist or their primary care provider. Therefore, it is likely that non-oncologists will be increasingly engaged in longitudinal care of breast cancer survivors.

This book is divided into sections to make it as easy as possible to find the information you need, whether it is related to basic breast health or breast cancer prevention, screening, treatment, or survivorship. The authors are members of the Johns Hopkins University School of Medicine faculty and staff who specialize in the assessment, diagnosis, treatment, and prevention of breast cancer.

Once a patient's treatment is completed, she will be seen less frequently by members of her breast cancer medical team but will always be returning to see you. Our goal for this book is to provide non-cancer specialists and their patients with the necessary information to ensure continuity of care, to optimize general health, and to reduce the risk of breast cancer recurrence.

Nancy Davidson, MD
Director of Breast Cancer Research
Johns Hopkins Breast Center

Introduction

A great deal of thought and consideration was given to deciding what information should be contained in this book. We wanted to provide an easy-to-read guide to assist health care providers in the fields of gynecology, internal medicine, and primary care in the monitoring and long-term management of women with various types of breast health issues, especially breast cancer.

Currently 77% of women diagnosed with breast cancer are age 50 or older; however, it is projected that approximately 66% of the new cases diagnosed will occur in women younger than 65.[1] We have seen and treated a large number of young women at Johns Hopkins in recent years and have certainly seen a growing number of young women entering our Breast Center doors. No doubt you have seen an increase in the incidence of the disease among your own patients in addition to perhaps their age group getting younger. Breast cancer is no longer considered a disease of older women.

Because of the increased incidence of this disease, you can anticipate seeing your patients—and in some cases, patients new to your practice—turning to you to serve as their "breast cancer survivor doctor." As mentioned in the Preface of this text, an article in the *Journal of Clinical Oncology*, Vol. 24, No. 6, Feb 20, 2006, entitled *Randomized Trial of Long-Term Follow-up for Early Stage Breast Cancer—A Comparison of Family Physician vs Specialist Care*, confirms that survival is equal for patients, whether followed long-term by their oncologist, gynecologist, or primary care provider. Family practitioners, internal medicine doctors, and gynecologists, as well as nurse practioners in these fields, however, may not have the necessary knowledge to appropriately and confidently follow breast cancer patients. The pressure to do so, and the expectations of the primary care physician (PCP) and others involved in the field of women's health, will escalate with the confirmation that it is safe to do and with the need for oncologists to transfer their long-term patients to PCPs in order to make room for the additional volume of newly diagnosed patients coming in the near future. Statistics for 2007 predict 178,480 women and 2,030 men will be diagnosed with invasive breast cancer in the United States along with 44,030 individuals diagnosed with DCIS, noninvasive breast cancer, and an estimated 41,000 people will die.[2] With baby boomers coming into midlife, these numbers will continue to grow. Primary care providers, gynecologists, and other health care professionals will play an increasingly important role in the monitoring and care of breast cancer survivors after treatment is completed. Therefore PCPs, based on their role in health maintenance and disease prevention, are best positioned to address the full spectrum of cancer survivor health needs, provided they are empowered with the information they need to confidently manage their patients' long-term follow-up care.

Some health care providers may not be familiar with the clinical assessment and diagnostic steps needed to evaluate patients with a breast health problem, or even with the optimum time to refer patients for additional work-up at a comprehensive breast center. A delay in the diagnosis of breast cancer remains a leading cause of medical malpractice today.

The information contained in this book is intended to provide the knowledge you need as a primary health care provider involved with women's health, with a specific focus on breast health and breast cancer. This book contains information related to the types of technology used today for diagnosing breast health problems, both benign and malignant; assisting your patients in understanding their treatment options related to breast cancer surgical management; the newest techniques for breast reconstruction; the various protocols available for chemotherapy, radiation therapy, targeted therapy, and hormonal therapy; and the many side effects that your patients may have to deal with during and following completion of their treatment. A special focus has been given to addressing the medical needs and psychological well-being of the breast cancer patient after her adjuvant therapy is finished. She will be seeing you more often and seeing her oncology team less frequently, and, in many cases, perhaps not seeing a cancer specialist at all . . . acknowledging *you* as the breast cancer survivor doctor.

The chapters are in a specific order to walk you through the process of how to select a Breast Center or breast specialists qualified to address the patient's needs, the diagnostic tools available and when and who should order them, the patient's breast cancer treatment across the continuum, your important role after treatment is completed to help maintain her health and survivorship, and even information related to assessing the patient and her family for possibly having a genetic predisposition to developing breast cancer. We have provided a breast pathology chapter that answers questions about virtually any type of pathology result that you may receive from a breast biopsy or surgical specimen and how to interpret it. Pharmacogenetics information is provided as well, given that patients can be on a variety of additional medications unrelated to their breast cancer treatment that may negatively influence the effectiveness of prescribed cancer treatments. In addition, there is also a special chapter on participation in clinical trials and why it is important to discuss participation with your patients. Furthermore, you will find evidence-based medicine that supports ways to reduce your patient's side effects related to short- and long-term treatment, for which she will seek your assistance. There is also specific information about the importance of helping patients maintain compliance with their treatment, particularly hormonal therapy that needs to be taken for several years after other treatment has ended.

This book contains a variety of algorithms, charts, medical illustrations, and photographs as well as a frequently asked questions (FAQ) section at the end of each chapter. These are intended to provide you with a quick reference for specific information that you may need, and supporting documentation within the context of the chapter.

As an additional aid for you and your patients, we have provided a resource chapter in the back of this book. It contains a list of credible organizations that provide educational information and support to patients and their families who are journeying through breast cancer treatment.

We hope that you find this book helpful in your clinical practice as we share the challenge of taking care of women with breast health problems, especially those diagnosed in the future with breast cancer.

Lillie D. Shockney

REFERENCES

1. http://www.cancer.gov
2. http://www.cancer.gov/cancertopics/types/breast

Editors

Lillie D. Shockney, RN, BS, MAS
Administrative Director, Johns Hopkins Avon Foundation Breast Center
Assistant Professor of Surgery and Gynecology

Mrs. Shockney is a registered nurse with a BS in Health Care Administration from Saint Joseph's College and a Masters in Administrative Science from Johns Hopkins University. She has worked at Johns Hopkins since 1983 and has served as the Administrative Director since 1997. As Administrative Director she is responsible for the quality of care programs; patient education programs; the survivor volunteer team; community outreach at the local, regional, and national levels; webmaster, and patient advocacy.

Mrs. Shockney has written six books and more than 90 articles on breast cancer and is a nationally recognized public speaker on the subject. She serves on the medical advisory board of several national breast cancer organizations and is the co-founder and vice president of a national non-profit organization called "Mothers Supporting Daughters with Breast Cancer."

She is also the recipient of the Global Business Leadership award, numerous community service awards, was the recipient of the Outstanding Women of America Award, in 1997 was awarded the Distinguished Graduate for Lifetime Achievement Award, and in 1998 received the National Silver Medal Award from the National Consumer Health Information Center. In 1999 she was the recipient of the National Circle of Life Award and the American Cancer Society's Voice of Hope Award; in 2001, she was the recipient of the ACS Lane Adams Award for Excellence in Caring; in 2000, she was selected as an "Unsung Hero" for breast cancer by Pharmacia & Upjohn's 2001 calendar.

She also received the 2001 Lane A. Adams Award for Excellence in Caring from the American Cancer Society. In addition Mrs. Shockney has received the 2002 Faces of Breast Cancer, ACS, and the 2002 Oncology Nursing Society Award for Excellence in Breast Cancer Education awards. In 2003 she was the recipient of the Impact Award from the National Consortium of Breast Centers. She was also the recipient of the Komen Award from the Maryland Affiliate in 2003. In 2004 she was a finalist for the Lance Armstrong Foundation's Spirit of Survivorship award and was selected as one of the Top 100 Women in Maryland for her leadership and community service efforts. Mrs. Shockney was selected by the Komen Foundation, nationally, to receive the 2005 Professor of Survivorship Award. In 2006 she was the recipient of the Spirit of Friends Award from Food & Friends and the Avon Foundation, and also received the Patient of Courage Award from the American Plastic Surgery Society. Mrs. Shockney was the recipient of the 2007 Yoplait Breast Cancer Champion award. Her research focus is in the area of quality of life research.

Theodore (Ted) N. Tsangaris, MD
Medical Director of the Johns Hopkins Avon Foundation Breast Center
Chief of Breast Surgery
Associate Professor of Surgery

Dr. Tsangaris joined the Johns Hopkins faculty in March 2002 as the Medical Director of the Johns Hopkins Breast Center and Chief of Breast Surgery, Division of Surgical Oncology. He earned his BA at Wake Forest University in 1979, was awarded his MD degree at George Washington University School of Medicine in 1983, and completed his General Surgery Residency at George Washington University and his Surgical Breast Oncology Fellowship at Baylor University Medical Center in 1990. He attended Harvard School of Public Health and Harvard School of Medicine during the summer of 1994, where he completed their educational program in Clinical Effectiveness. An accomplished surgical oncologist who specializes in breast cancer, he has held several leadership positions prior to joining the Johns Hopkins faculty. These include Assistant Professor and Acting Chief of Breast Surgery at Roswell Park Cancer Institute in New York from 1990–1992; Visiting Surgical Consultant for the

Saudi–US University Project for King Faisal Specialist Hospital and Research Center in Saudi Arabia from 1995–1997; Director, Student Clerkships in the Department of Surgery at George Washington University Medical Center during 1995–1997, and Assistant Professor of Surgery and Director of the Breast Cancer Center at George Washington University from 1993–1997. From 1997 to February 2002, he was the Director of Breast Surgical Services and Associate Professor of Surgery at Lombardi Cancer Center at the Georgetown University's Medical Center in Washington, DC.

Dr. Tsangaris is a nationally renowned breast surgical oncologist with expertise in surgical management as well as a breadth of knowledge and experience in clinical research in the field of breast cancer.

Contributors

Pedram Argani, MD
Director of Breast Pathology
Associate Professor of Pathology

Dr. Argani is a graduate of the University of Pennsylvania School of Medicine and received his pathology training at the Hospital of the University of Pennsylvania in Philadelphia. He also completed fellowships in Oncologic Pathology and Molecular Pathology at Memorial Sloan-Kettering Cancer Center in New York, where he studied under the guidance of such noted pathologists as Dr. Juan Rosai, Dr. Paul Peter Rosen, and Dr. Marc Ladanyl. Dr. Argani is board certified in Anatomic Pathology.

Dr. Argani first joined the Johns Hopkins Pathology faculty in 1997, and is now an Associate Professor of Pathology at Johns Hopkins University School of Medicine and Attending Pathologist at Johns Hopkins Hospital where he is also Director of Breast Pathology. His major areas of interest are the diagnostic pathology and molecular pathogenesis of breast cancer, particularly through the characterization of new markers of cancer. At the 2007 United States and Canadian Academy of Pathology meeting, Dr. Argani received the Arthur Purdy Stout Society prize, given annually to a Surgical Pathologist under the age of 45 in recognition of career research achievements. Dr. Argani routinely reviews slides from patients with breast tumors who are treated at Johns Hopkins, in order to provide a second opinion. To arrange for this review, please contact the Anatomic Pathology Consultation Office at Johns Hopkins Hospital, (410) 955-2405. This office is located at 1620 McElderry Street, Reed Hall, Room 315, Baltimore, MD 21205, fax (410) 614-7712.

Deborah K. Armstrong, MD
Director of BOSS Program
Associate Professor of Oncology, Gynecology and Obstetrics

Dr. Armstrong received her bachelor's degree in bacteriology from the University of California at Berkeley and then attended the George Washington University School of Medicine. While at George Washington, she was elected to the Alpha Omega Alpha medical honor society and was awarded the American Medical Women's Association Scholarship Achievement Citation. Dr. Armstrong received her MD degree with distinction and then completed training in internal medicine at the University of Pittsburgh and served as Chief Medical Resident. Dr. Armstrong trained in medical oncology as a fellow at the Johns Hopkins Oncology Center. During her oncology training, Dr. Armstrong was awarded fellowships from the Susan G. Komen Foundation and the Stetler Research Fund. Since joining the Johns Hopkins faculty, Dr. Armstrong has received a Young Investigator Award from the American Society of Clinical Oncology, a *Ladies Home Journal* Breakthrough Achievement Award, and has twice received the Johns Hopkins University Department of Medicine Osler Housestaff Teaching Award.

Dr. Armstrong works primarily in the area of women's malignancies, with a particular emphasis on breast cancer, ovarian cancer, and other gynecologic malignancies, and the genetics of breast and ovarian cancer. Dr. Armstrong's clinical focus is on the development of new therapeutic approaches to the treatment of breast cancer and gynecologic malignancies. Particular areas of interest are intraperitoneal therapy, targeted biologic therapy, and immunologic approaches to cancer treatment. Dr. Armstrong also directs the Johns Hopkins Breast and Ovarian Cancer Screening Service, a genetic counseling service that focuses on identifying patients at risk for cancer and examination of new strategies for cancer screening and prevention.

Charles Balch, MD
Professor of Surgery and Oncology

Dr. Balch has been a Professor of Surgery and Oncology at Johns Hopkins since 2000. He has been a surgical oncologist for over 30 years, specializing clinically in breast cancer and melanoma. He received his medical degree at Columbia College of Physicians and Surgeons. Dr. Balch was trained in surgery at Duke Medical Center and the University of Alabama at Birmingham. He also completed a fellowship in immunology at Scripps Clinic and Research Foundation.

Dr. Balch has published over 560 scientific articles, book chapters, and abstracts, including numerous scientific articles and book chapters specifically about breast cancer. He was the founding Editor-in-Chief of the journal "Breast Diseases" as well as the founding Editor-in-Chief of *The Annals of Surgical Oncology*. He has held numerous leadership roles including Executive Vice-President and CEO of the American Society of Clinical Oncology; President and CEO of the City of Hope National Medical Center; Chief of Surgery and Anesthesiology, Vice-President of Hospital and Clinics, and Executive Vice-President for Health Affairs at the University of Texas MD Anderson Cancer Center; and Chief of Surgical Oncology, Associate Director and Acting Director of the Comprehensive Cancer Center at the University of Alabama in Birmingham. He also has been President of the Association for Academic Surgery and the Society of Surgical Oncology and Chair of the Commission on Cancer for the American College of Surgeons. Dr. Balch is the recipient of the Society of Surgical Oncology's Heritage Award, 2006.

Nancy Davidson, MD
Director of the Breast Cancer Research Program at Johns Hopkins
Professor of Oncology

Dr. Davidson received her MD in 1979 from Harvard Medical School in Boston, Massachusetts, and completed internal medicine training at the Hospital of the University of Pennsylvania and Johns Hopkins. Dr. Davidson was a Medical Staff Fellow and guest worker at the National Cancer Institute in Bethesda, Maryland, from 1982–1986, where she developed a major interest in the breast cancer field. Dr. Davidson joined the faculty at the Johns Hopkins University School of Medicine in 1986 as a Professor of Oncology. Today Dr. Davidson is an Associate Professor of Oncology and Breast Cancer Research Chair in Oncology. She also serves as Director of the Breast Cancer Research Program.

Trained as a medical oncologist and scientist, Dr. Davidson has devoted her career to breast cancer research, both in the clinical and laboratory settings. Her clinical research has focused on the value of combination therapy with chemotherapy and hormonal therapy for young women with breast cancer. She has taken a leadership role in conducting national clinical trials for breast cancer. One of her major laboratory interests has been the definition of the biochemical pathways by which breast cancer cells die, with the hope that new targets for anti-breast cancer therapy can be identified.

Dr. Davidson is the 2007–2008 President of the American Society of Clinical Oncology.

Leisha A. Emens, MD, PhD
Assistant Professor of Oncology

Dr. Emens received her BA in Biochemistry and Cell Biology from the University of California at San Diego in 1984. She trained in the Medical Scientist Training Program at Baylor College of Medicine, receiving her PhD in Cell Biology in 1993, and her MD in 1995. She completed her internship and residency in internal medicine at the University of Texas at Southwestern Medical School in 1998. Dr. Emens came to the Johns Hopkins Hospital in 1998 and completed fellowship training in medical oncology and hematology in 2001. She joined the faculty at the Johns Hopkins University School of Medicine in 2001 as an Assistant Professor of Oncology. Dr. Emens is board-certified in internal medicine and medical oncology by the American Board of Internal Medicine, and her clinical interest in oncology is breast cancer. Dr. Emens has committed her career to the development of novel biologic therapies for breast cancer treatment and prevention, with an emphasis on vaccine- and monoclonal antibody-based immunotherapies. With formal training in both laboratory science and clinical medicine, her research is focused on testing immunotherapies and gene transfer technologies in clinical trials, and analyzing patient responses in the laboratory to identify new and pivotal immune and biologic targets for therapy. Dr. Emens is a member of the American Society of Clinical Oncology, the American Association for Cancer Research, and the American Society for Gene Therapy.

Nagi F. Khouri, MD
Director, Johns Hopkins Breast Imaging
Associate Professor of Radiology

Dr. Khouri earned his MD degree from the American University of Beirut in 1971. Following his residency training at Johns Hopkins in 1975, he was board certified in radiology and joined the full-time faculty as a chest radiologist from 1976 to 1986, where he was the head of that section. His clinical interests and research focused on lung cancer, computer tomography (CT) of the pulmonary nodule, and percutaneous lung biopsies. Since 1986, he has focused all of his efforts on the field of Breast Imaging and Intervention, first at the Diagnostic Breast Center of Cross Keys and later as the Director of Breast Imaging at Johns Hopkins at Green Spring-Station. His major areas of interest are breast imaging and intervention with a patient-oriented approach, breast ultrasound, and digital mammography. In 2007 he was recognized as one of the top five breast imaging specialists in the country.

Carol B. Riley, RN, MSN, CRNP
Oncology Nurse

Ms. Riley received her BSN from Towson State University in 1987. She then began working in the Oncology Center at Johns Hopkins in a solid tumor/bone marrow transplant unit. After eight years as a senior clinical nurse, Carol pursued her graduate program at Johns Hopkins University. She graduated in 1998 and obtained her Nurse Practitioner certification. Carol began working in the Breast Center with the medical oncology group in October of 1998. Carol provides support, education, and medical care for patients receiving drug treatments; including chemotherapy, hormonal therapies, and biologic therapies.

Dr. Gedge Rosson, MD
Director of Breast Plastic Surgery
Assistant Professor of Plastic and Reconstructive Surgery

Dr. Rosson graduated from New York Medical College in 1998 after receiving his undergraduate degree from the University of California,

Berkeley. He did his internship, general surgery, and plastic surgery residency training at Johns Hopkins Hospital. Dr. Rosson then completed a Peripheral Nerve Surgery Fellowship at the Dellon Institute for Peripheral Nerve Surgery in Baltimore, Maryland.

He is board certified by the American Board of Plastic Surgery and his academic appointments include Assistant Professor, Plastic Surgery at the Johns Hopkins University School of Medicine, and Clinical Assistant Professor at the University of Maryland.

He specializes in microvascular perforator flap breast reconstructions, such as the DIEP (deep inferior epigastric artery perforator flap), the SIEA (superficial inferior epigastric artery flap), and the SGAP (superior gluteal artery perforator flap). He was the first surgeon in the United States to widely implement pre-operative mapping of the abdominal perforators using 64-slice multi-detector 3D CT scan angiograms and he is one of the first to now regularly connect nerves to create sensate breast reconstructions.

Dr. Rosson currently has hospital privileges at Johns Hopkins Hospital, the R. Adams Cowley Shock-Trauma Center, and Union Memorial Hospital in Baltimore, Maryland. His research has been published in major peer-reviewed scientific journals and presented at both national and international meetings.

Navin Singh, MD
Diplomate, American Board of Plastic Surgery
Director of Resident Cosmetic Surgery Education
Assistant Professor of Plastic Surgery
Email: doctor@surgicalpoetry.com

Dr. Singh earned his medical degree at Brown University School of Medicine and his master's degree in Clinical Biostatistics at Harvard School of Public Health. He completed an internship in general surgery and a residency in plastic surgery at Johns Hopkins Hospital. Dr. Singh is a plastic surgeon at Johns Hopkins Hospital and is in private practice in Bethesda and Chevy Chase, Maryland. He is involved in several research efforts, with a concentration in breast reconstruction, perforator flaps such as DIEPs and SGAPs, and robot-assisted microsurgery, topics for which he also has published extensively and made numerous media appearances. He is the past Residency Program Director and past Director of Breast Reconstruction at Johns Hopkins.

A member of numerous professional societies, including the American Society for Aesthetic Plastic Surgery, the American Society of Plastic Surgeons, the International Trauma Anesthesia & Critical Care Society, and the American Society for Reconstructive Microsurgery, Dr. Singh has twice been the recipient of the Teacher of the Year award at Johns Hopkins and has been voted among America's Top Physicians and America's Top Plastic Surgeons by the Consumer Research Council of America. He was also the recipient of the "Hero Award" from the University of Maryland R. Adams Cowley Shock-Trauma Center in 2001.

Dr. Singh is on the editorial boards of the *Aesthetic Surgery Journal* and *Microsurgery* and is the plastic surgery advisor for the Breast Health Center of the National Women's Health Resource Center. Dr. Singh is an Assistant Professor in Surgery (Plastic) and has honorary appointments as Assistant Professor in Gynecology and in Neurosurgery because of his notable expertise and collaborative research in those fields.

Kala Visvanathan MD, MHS
Assistant Professor of Epidemiology and Oncology

Dr. Visvanathan received her medical degree from the University of Sydney in Australia. She subsequently went on to complete her training in Internal Medicine and Medical Oncology at Royal Prince Alfred, a teaching hospital of the University of Sydney, and the Sidney Kimmel Comprehensive Cancer Center at Johns Hopkins. In addition, she undertook a Masters in Clinical/Cancer epidemiology at the Johns Hopkins Bloomberg School of Public Health. Dr. Visvanathan currently has a joint faculty appointment in the Johns Hopkins School of Medicine and the Bloomberg School of Public Health. She is one of two physicians who run the high-risk breast and ovarian clinic at Johns Hopkins in addition to seeing cancer patients. Trained as a medical oncologist and cancer epidemiologist, Dr. Visvanathan's primary research interest is in the etiology, early detection, and prevention of breast and ovarian cancer. In particular, the evaluation of genetic, molecular, and dietary biomarkers of risk and early detection in breast cancer incidence and mortality, with an aim to modify those factors in the causal pathway with effective chemoprevention strategies.

Richard Zellars, MD
Assistant Professor Radiation Oncology

Dr. Zellars graduated from the Johns Hopkins School of Medicine in 1991. He did a one-year internship at Greater Baltimore Medical Center; his residency at the University of Michigan Medical Center in the Department of Radiation Oncology, where he was Chief Resident from 1995–1996; and was Assistant Professor/Vice-Chair and Clinic Director at the University of Texas Health Science Center at San Antonio for three and a half years. Prior to coming to Johns Hopkins he was Assistant Professor at Georgetown University. Dr. Zellars' primary area of interest is carcinoma of the breast. Dr. Zellars is listed as one of the top doctors for women by both *Redbook* and *Ladies Home Journal*. His grant-supported research aims to provide safety, facility, and efficacy of radiation.

Algorithm for Selecting a Breast Center

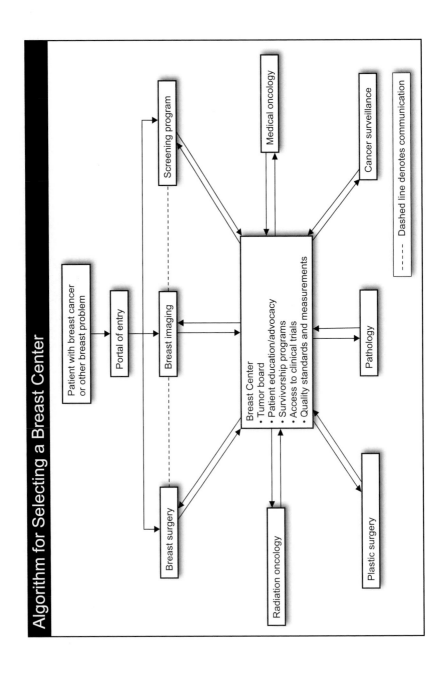

chapter

1

Selecting a Breast Center to Refer Patients

Lillie D. Shockney, RN, BS, MAS

What you need to know:

Not all facilities that call themselves a "Breast Center" qualify for the title. Seek a facility that is part of a National Cancer Institute (NCI)–designated comprehensive cancer center whenever possible.

You're responsible for providing the consulting physician at the Breast Center with the pertinent medical information that explains your findings on the patient's clinical exam, as well as her medical history and other significant information that reflects the purpose of the consultation. If you are a primary care provider (PCP), be sure that the necessary referrals are provided to expedite her being seen.

Be sure that the facility and health care providers you select for your patient do the following:

▷ Provide easy access and prompt appointments

▷ Promote patient education and participation

▷ Offer a multidisciplinary approach to care and treatment, including having a breast cancer tumor board for case presentation and team discussion

▷ Preferably offer minimally invasive diagnostic methods over surgical methods for assessing and determining a diagnosis

▷ Preferably offer digital mammography (instead of just standard analog mammography)

▷ Provide you with feedback about the outcome of the consultation and communicate well with you and your office staff

▷ Offer innovative care including access and participation in clinical trials

▷ Provide state-of-the-art surgical options including all forms of breast reconstruction

▷ Be board certified in their specialty and specialize in breast cancer; this includes the breast surgeon, medical oncologist, radiation oncologist, mammographer, and pathologist

▷ Offer high-risk assessment and genetics counseling

▷ Address urgent care needs of your patient promptly and effectively during her treatment

▷ Provide your patient with support services to address her emotional well-being during and after treatment

▷ Demonstrate that the facility and all aspects of the care it renders are measured from the perspective of clinical quality outcomes

Ask your patient for feedback during her experience as well as after her consultations and treatment are completed at the Breast Center you have selected for her.

What your patient needs to know:

The patient cannot judge a Breast Center's credentials based on the facility's (paid) advertisements in the media. She needs to rely on you for direction. It requires a lot of effort for her to do the necessary due diligence to ensure she is in good hands. Your input should be requested and relied upon when selecting where she goes for breast health care.

She should provide you with feedback about how her experience was at the Breast Center.

She is responsible for following the instructions given regarding what to bring with her or where to send these items in advance of her visit there. This might include pathology slides from a biopsy performed, mammogram images (not just the report), and copies of your medical records.

The patient also needs information from you as to why you selected the physician/Breast Center you are sending her to for evaluation. Tell her what the features are that you felt were important in making this decision on her behalf.

INTRODUCTION

One of the challenges today for clinicians is deciding where to refer patients with a breast problem, particularly breast cancer. It is easy to tell a patient to go to a "Breast Center"; unfortunately there are no standards that define what is meant by this term. Those of us who have worked in this field for decades believe we know what the features, services, and standards of care should be, but these are not universally applied or understood. However, you want to make sure that your patient is in good hands and that her breast health needs will be appropriately and efficiently addressed. You probably already have a working relationship with specific surgeons, radiologists, oncologists, and others. These may be well-established relationships that have been fostered over a period of years. This may be a time to revisit those relationships and gain a better understanding of what your patients' needs are and who is best to address them.

Perhaps you refer patients to Radiologist X in the suburbs for mammography and ultrasound but to Breast Surgeon Z, who works in the city at a teaching hospital. Many health care professionals would say that ideally you would refer a patient to one center that has a multidisciplinary team, where whatever her needs are they can be addressed in one location by specialists who work together professionally and who you know are good: a Breast Center that is part of a National Cancer Institute (NCI)–designated comprehensive cancer center. There are certainly situations in which your patient may not need a facility offering all of the services and programs that are part of such a center. For example, she may simply need a good diagnostic evaluation in an accredited breast imaging facility. However, having fostered relationships with health care professionals who are part of a larger entity can be helpful for you as well as for your patients. The following are some points to consider when making such decisions on your patients' behalf.

EASY ACCESS

If your patient has been diagnosed with breast cancer or there is a strong suspicion that this is the diagnosis, you will want an appointment for her as soon as possible. That is not because it is a medical emergency but rather because until she has a plan of action the patient will feel anxious, out of control, and in a state of limbo. You want her taken care of in a timely manner. Most Breast Centers, in acknowledgment of this, will (and should) schedule your patient for an appointment within 72 hours of your call to make the referral. This would entail either having her into breast imaging for diagnostic evaluation/work-up so a diagnosis can be made, or seeing a breast surgeon if she is already diagnosed with breast cancer. In some cases, the breast surgeon sees the patient prior to obtaining a core biopsy to gain clinical information through the clinical breast exam (CBE), then refers her for diagnostic evaluation and biopsy. It is helpful to know which critical pathway is preferred based on where you are referring the patient.

PATIENT EMPOWERMENT

Patients deserve to be empowered so that they can actively participate in decisions about their care and treatment. Some physicians are reluctant to empower women in this way. It is a patient's right and should be a key factor in deciding where you want her to receive her treatment. Seek a health care team that specializes in breast diseases and breast cancer so that this is one of the services offered. Based on patient satisfaction studies done here at Johns Hopkins, the more we empower a patient and give her a solid knowledge base about her breast issue, the more satisfied she is with her care. That should also translate into her being happy with you and your choice in where you referred her to obtain that breast care. This also includes educating other family members when appropriate.[1]

MULTIDISCIPLINARY TUMOR BOARD/CASE CONFERENCES

A key advantage to having a multidisciplinary team approach is the special expertise each health care professional offers given each patient's unique situation. Centers that hold weekly breast cancer case conferences (sometimes referred to as "breast cancer tumor boards") to discuss in detail a patient's clinical condition, diagnostic findings, and recommendations for optimal treatment, are beneficial to the patient's overall well-being and clinical outcome. This is a way to help ensure that the patient is being given individualized attention and care by utilizing maximum breast cancer knowledge, experience, and expertise by the Breast Center team. All NCI-designated cancer centers are required to conduct such conferences on a regular basis and maintain records of the cases presented. Usually the patient is informed by the physician presenting her case that her clinical situation is going to be discussed by the team. The physician then gets back to the patient to inform her of the discussion and outcome of that presentation.[2]

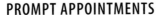

PROMPT APPOINTMENTS

If a woman is being referred by her family doctor or gynecologist for evaluation of a suspicious lump or other potentially serious breast abnormality (such as a newly inverted nipple), she wants to know right away if it is cancer. For that matter, if she finds the lump herself, she does not want there to be any delay in getting answers about her situation. Mammography facilities should offer appointments for such patients as quickly as possible. Ideally the patient would be seen within 2 to 3 days of the referral being made by you. Often radiologists are not readily available to read the films and talk with the patient about what the mammogram showed. It is important to refer your patient to a facility that has radiologists who specialize in breast imaging and are available to read the films while she is there, and, most importantly, tell her what they show. Having the radiologist give you rapid feedback regarding the results is also key. Some breast imaging facilities will proceed in doing additional diagnostic evaluation based on the results of the preliminary findings—for example, if they think an ultrasound is needed, it is done at that time rather than scheduling another appointment. If a biopsy is needed, it is obtained immediately, again reducing the patient's anxiety by getting answers more swiftly, including getting back to you with the diagnosis.

MINIMALLY INVASIVE STEREOTACTIC BREAST BIOPSY, CORE BIOPSY, AND FINE-NEEDLE BIOPSIES

Several types of biopsy procedures can be done in the breast imaging facility, thereby enabling a rapid pathology result and avoiding an incision, general anesthesia, and, in general, scarring inside the breast that may appear as abnormalities on future mammograms. Some facilities do a high volume of these types of procedures; others may not. In general, studies demonstrate that the more procedures you do, the better you are in general at doing that procedure. Radiologists who specialize in breast imaging and diagnostic evaluation along with diagnostic interventions are important for a patient undergoing such a procedure. There have been many patients who have come to our doors having been told elsewhere that they need an open surgical biopsy when, in fact, the biopsy can be obtained in a minimally invasive manner. Today more than 90% of biopsies can be obtained in this manner, typically with results from pathology by the next business day.

DIGITAL MAMMOGRAPHY

Research studies have confirmed that women who are premenopausal and have dense breast tissue on (analog film) mammography can benefit by having their mammogram captured digitally as a computer image. Digital mammography is not available everywhere yet, and it will likely be several years before it is, due to the equipment being expensive. Patients are becoming more knowledgeable, however, and are seeking out facilities themselves where digital mammography is available. You can aid them by finding out what Breast Centers and breast imaging facilities have this capability and how long it has been in place.[3]

GETTING INFORMATION BACK TO YOU ABOUT THE OUTCOME OF THE REFERRAL

There is probably nothing more frustrating to you than sending a patient to another provider and then not knowing what happened. Find out the other provider's method of communication for providing you with prompt feedback regarding your patient. Does the provider have a system in place whereby the transition is smooth? Once you refer the patient, is the other provider able to take care of the rest of her breast health needs, or does the patient need to return to you for additional referral decisions? You may prefer that the patient return to you after her consultative referral is completed or you may want the Breast Center to do diagnostic evaluation, provide a diagnosis, transfer her to a breast surgeon if needed, and continue her on her clinical pathway for treatment. The doctors taking care of her need to keep you in the loop, however, so making them aware of how this process will happen and how you want it to occur is important. Give them feedback if it is not working in the manner in which you expect.

CLINICAL TRIALS

Having the opportunity to have available to your patients as many treatment options as possible can be valuable. Breast Centers that participate in clinical trials can usually offer more innovative treatment options. Participation in a clinical trial offers your patient treatment that is at a minimum as good as the standard of care and may be better than current standards of care. If she is asked to participate in such a trial, the patient is also paving the way for the development of innovative research that will make an important impact on other women diagnosed in the future with breast cancer. She is also being closely monitored throughout her treatment process so that data can be collected about her experience with the chemotherapy agents she's receiving.

FULL RANGE OF SURGICAL OPTIONS: STATE-OF-THE-ART BREAST CANCER SURGERY

It is unfortunate that in medical school breast cancer surgery is treated as a simple procedure. However, if you were the patient and it was your breast, you might not consider it quite so simple. It is very important for breast cancer surgery to be performed by a surgeon who has chosen breast cancer surgery as his or her surgical specialty and who does a large volume of breast cancer surgeries on an annual basis. (Note I said breast *cancer* surgeries—not breast surgeries.) It is preferable that the surgeon be a surgical oncologist who specializes in breast cancer. Such surgeons are generally found at large teaching hospitals, which are a part of comprehensive cancer centers. Published research studies confirm that breast surgeons who do a high volume of breast cancer surgeries have higher survival results than those who do not.[4, 5] There is also an expectation that such surgeons will maintain clinical quality outcomes data.

Ask what type of preoperative teaching is offered for patients and their families as well. Usually a Breast Center will have dedicated nurses to provide education to patients so that they are well prepared for the type of surgery they are to have, thereby reducing anxiety prior to and at the time of surgery.

More than 80% of women are good candidates for breast conservation surgery today, especially those with stage 1 or 2 unifocal breast cancer. Sentinel node biopsy is also currently the standard of care, enabling the surgeon to identify the guard node and remove only that single node to determine if the cancer has spread. This has dramatically reduced the risk of lymphedema, a major concern for women having axillary node dissections.

Women needing mastectomy or desiring this as their surgical option also have the right to a full spectrum of reconstruction options. Not all options are available at all Breast Centers, however. A patient may need to travel elsewhere for other reconstruction procedures, such as deep inferior epigastric perforator (DIEP) flap or superior gluteal artery perforator (S-GAP) surgeries, which require microvascular surgery to rebuild the breast. These reconstruction methods combined with skin-sparing mastectomy offer women cosmetic results far superior to what was available in past years. They also reduce the risk of hernia, bulge, and other complications more commonly found with transverse rectus abdominus myocutaneous (TRAM) flap surgeries. Again you want your patient in the hands of a plastic surgeon who has done a large volume of the type of reconstruction from which the patient would most benefit. These surgeons also would be maintaining clinical outcomes data and should have available at the time of the patient's consultation "before and after" photographs that show her each type of reconstruction option.

MEDICAL ONCOLOGY

Your patient will feel more confident being treated by a medical oncologist who specializes in breast cancer than a general medical oncologist who treats a variety of oncologic diseases. Someone who treats a large number of women with this disease and has access to a spectrum of clinical trials for her are other factors to consider. Even if a patient doesn't need chemotherapy, commonly she is still referred to a medical oncologist for discussion about adjuvant therapy, including possibly being a candidate for hormonal therapy.

Ask about the physician's office practice for handling emergent issues that may arise for your patient, such as being febrile or having uncontrolled nausea and vomiting, so that you are confident that she is being managed well.

Ask about what education is available to help your patient prepare for known side effects of treatment. Inquire about how patients are referred for wig fittings as well as skin care needs that may occur during treatment. Some Breast Centers offer these services within their facilities.

Targeted therapy is now available, and more forms of targeted therapy will be developed in the near future. For patients who have a specific prognostic factor, an oncogene called HER2/neu-receptor positivity, the medical oncologist may recommend targeted therapy in the form of trastuzumab (Herceptin). This therapy is commonly administered for approximately one year.

RADIATION ONCOLOGY

Most patients who have breast conservation surgery or who have locally advanced disease will probably be advised to undergo radiation therapy in some manner. Again, it is valuable to use a facility that has extensive experience with treating this specific type of cancer. The center will have a physicist on staff who assists with the treatment planning. There are currently different methods of delivering radiation for breast cancer treatment. Some are part of clinical trials and some are standards of care. Patients will want to know how their heart and lungs will be protected from the radiation field. A device called Active Breath Control Device is available at some centers that provides a more reliable way for the patient's heart and lungs to be spared radiation by controlling breathing during the actual radiation treatment.[6]

GENETIC COUNSELING AND HIGH-RISK ASSESSMENT

Having a patient evaluated for risk of developing breast cancer or a family member getting this disease is something that will probably start in your office and then result in a referral to a formal genetics evaluation specialist. High-risk assessment, counseling, and genetic testing require specialists who are not only experts in this field but who also have excellent communication skills. The choice to have counseling and, especially, to decide to proceed with genetic testing is one to be taken seriously and with some caution. Although it can sound simple to be tested, there are many things to consider before proceeding with genetic testing. Ask how long the program has existed and how many patients have been counseled and tested during that time. This will give you some idea as to the provider's experience with this specialized type of service. The genetics test itself is not done on site. It is sent to one laboratory in the United States that performs this test. If a woman tests positive for a *BRCA* gene, she will need professional help in deciding how she wants to approach prevention—some patients will decide to do prophylactic mastectomies, whereas others may opt to take hormonal therapy or simply undergo close monitoring. Therefore, the assessment of such a program for your patients needs to include which services and programs are part of the genetics counseling and high-risk assessment process.

Also ask if the center offers a screening–prevention program for patients who fall into the "worried well" group or who have high-risk factors that warrant being seen more often than annually for a clinical breast exam and mammogram. Some facilities have specially trained teams of nurse practitioners fulfilling this role, under the supervision of a physician.

PATHOLOGY SERVICES

Patients don't always think about this particular service, but it is a very important one. The pathologist who looks at your patient's tissue specimen determines the staging and prognostic factors, which results in the rest of the team using that information to formulate a treatment plan. Accuracy and completeness are critical. Some say that the pathologist "holds all the cards" because his or her opinion about what is on your patient's pathology slides is so critical. We don't want to overtreat or undertreat a patient, yet this happens every day across the United States because there are no clear standards regarding pathology interpretation. A Breast Center that has chosen to have pathologists who specialize in breast pathology has an edge, because these pathologists are likely to see higher volume than other pathologists, and they have made a commitment personally and professionally to specialize in breast disease.

CONTINUITY OF CARE

You need to have confidence on behalf of your patients that your patients are being watched over and cared for appropriately. Some facilities have nurse practitioners who stay in touch with patients via telephone once they are home from surgery and/or chemotherapy. Some offer home health nursing care after surgical treatment is complete. More are beginning to offer patient navigators to help with coordination of care. The members of the team of professionals taking care of your patient also need to stay in close contact with one another—that is why they are a team. Ask them how they communicate and keep each other informed about a patient's progress and needs. You want your patient cared for by a team that stays well connected with you, with one another, and with your patient. Feeling confident that your patient is receiving good continuity of care provides peace of mind to you, the patient, and her family.[7]

URGENT CARE NEEDS SERVICES

When an urgent medical problem arises such as vomiting that will not subside, clear processes of care need to be in place for patient management. Ask about the Breast Center's procedures for handling such emergencies. A Breast Center needs to have available for its patients a professional health care provider to handle emergencies, 24 hours a day, 7 days a week. In addition, patients should be well informed about how to access this urgent care service and know they can confidently rely on it. Although your patient may never need to use it, you want to know that such a program is in place and that it works well.

CONTINUING EDUCATION PROGRAMS AND SEMINARS

When her treatment is over, your patient will still want to stay up-to-date and informed regarding the latest treatment programs and research discoveries being made about breast cancer. Most patients thirst for information and want to learn as much as they can. Ask to be on the mailing list for these upcoming seminars and educational programs so that you can also share them with your patients. Also inquire about what continuing medical education (CME) programs are available related to breast disease and breast health that you may personally be interested in learning more about.

EMOTIONAL SUPPORT

Your patient needs to be treated as a total person. She is not just a stage 2b breast cancer patient. She is a school teacher, recently divorced, with two young children and a mother who has chronic illnesses and lives with her. Breast Centers usually provide social work counseling, breast cancer survivor volunteers for her to speak with, and nurses, along with others to help her as she navigates along her journey of treatment. Some centers, like ours, offer to match a newly diagnosed patient with a survivor volunteer based on her age, stage of disease, and anticipated treatment plan. Patients usually value the opportunity to talk with others who have made it through the process, building their confidence that they can do the same.

MEASURING QUALITY

Although the data may not yet be public, the pressure is mounting to develop national quality standards for the diagnosis and treatment of breast cancer. Several organizations are vigorously working on establishing quality measures and benchmarks for breast cancer care. A few include the American College of Surgeons, the National Consortium of Breast Centers, the National Quality Forum, the National Commission on Quality Assurance, and the National Comprehensive Care

Network. There are even movements afoot to look at developing a "pay for performance" process that would financially reward those Breast Centers that demonstrate high quality and good clinical outcomes. Watch for more information coming out in the media about this.[8]

SELECTING THE RIGHT TEAM FOR YOUR PATIENT

Selecting the right team for your patient also means selecting the right team for you. Who you refer your patients to reflects on you as well. Your patients are relying on you to choose well on their behalf. Asking questions like those listed in the previous pages lets the doctors and nurses who specialize in breast cancer and breast disease know that you are interested in ensuring that your patients are in the best possible hands.

∼ Frequently Asked Questions

1. *How should a patient go about selecting where she should go for her breast health assessment and/or breast cancer treatment?*

   It is common today to see commercials on television and advertisements in local magazines and newspapers promoting a specific Breast Center. However, this is not the method that your patient should be using to select where to go. She needs to rely to some degree on you for advice and expertise about where her care should be provided. Today it is becoming even more important than ever to ensure she is in good hands. A delayed diagnosis or mixed diagnosis of breast cancer can cost her not just her breast but her life. She needs to be in the hands of specialists—beginning with a radiologist who specializes in breast imaging and does a high volume of screening, diagnostic evaluation, and diagnostic intervention. If dealing with breast cancer, she needs a multidisciplinary team, all of whom specialize in this disease. She needs easy access to care, continuity of care that is seamless for her and that promotes her participation in the decision making about her treatment, as well as access to clinical trials that may give her an edge over standard therapy.

2. How do I as a physician go about finding out the details of what each Breast Center offers in my region?

Take the time to not just ask, but consider site visits, especially if you are in a field of medicine (like family practice and gynecology) in which you can anticipate and probably do see a large volume of women in need of breast health care. Use this chapter as your guide to know which questions to ask. Note the services and programs they offer. Ask about their volumes and quality measures. You want to ensure that your patients are in good hands.

REFERENCES

1. Melin M. Patient empowerment—the way forward. Eur J Cancer Care 1996;5(3 suppl):9.
2. Petit T. Mulitdisplinary approach in breast cancer care. Rev Prat 2004; 54:842–846.
3. Van Ongeval C, Bosmans H, Van Steen A, et al. Evaluation of the diagnostic value of a computed radiography system by comparison of digital hard copy images with screen film mammography: Results of a prospective clinical trial. Eur Radiol 2006;16:1360–1366.
4. Gillis CR, Hole David J. Survival outcome of care by specialist surgeons in breast cancer: A study of 3786 patients in the west of Scotland. BMJ 1996;312:145–148.
5. Allgood PC, Bachmann MO. Effects of specialization on treatment and outcomes in screening-detected breast cancers in Wales: Cohort study. Br J Cancer 2006;94:36–42.
6. Remouchamps VM, Letts N, Vicini FA, et al. Initial clinical experience with moderate deep-inspiration breath hold using an active breathing control device in the treatment of patients with left-sided breast cancer using external beam radiation therapy. Int J Radiat Oncol Biol Phys 2003;56:704–715.
7. Bairati I, et al. Women's perceptions of events impeding or facilitating the detection, investigation and treatment of breast cancer. Eur J Cancer Care 2006;15:183–193.
8. Grossbart SR. What's the return? Assessing the effect of "pay for performance" initiatives on the quality of care delivery. Med Care Res Rev 2006;63(1 suppl):29S–48S.

Algorithm for Breast Imaging

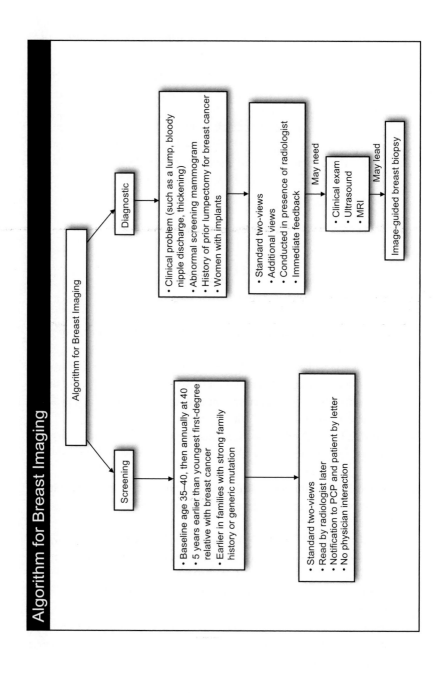

Algorithm for Breast Imaging

Screening

- Baseline age 35–40, then annually at 40
- 5 years earlier than youngest first-degree relative with breast cancer
- Earlier in families with strong family history or generic mutation

- Standard two-views
- Read by radiologist later
- Notification to PCP and patient by letter
- No physician interaction

Diagnostic

- Clinical problem (such as a lump, bloody nipple discharge, thickening)
- Abnormal screening mammogram
- History of prior lumpectomy for breast cancer
- Women with implants

- Standard two-views
- Additional views
- Conducted in presence of radiologist
- Immediate feedback

May need

- Clinical exam
- Ultrasound
- MRI

May lead

Image-guided breast biopsy

chapter

2

Diagnostic Evaluation/Image Guided Biopsies

Nagi F. Khouri, MD

What you need to know:

Screening mammography has reduced breast cancer mortality by 30% and in some studies by as much as 60% for women who have it performed annually.

Screening mammography criteria for you to follow with your patients are as follows:

▷ Women age 40 years and older should have it done annually; women age 80 years and older can have it done every other year.

▷ Women who have a first-degree relative diagnosed with breast cancer should begin mammography 5 years prior to the age of their relative was at time of diagnosis.

▷ Women with several first-degree relatives diagnosed with breast cancer should begin mammography 10 years prior to the youngest age of their relative at time of diagnosis; they may also need genetic counseling. Mammographic screening is rarely used for women younger than 30 years of age. Ultrasound is more commonly used for women in this age group for evaluation of a problem such as a lump.

Approximately 5% to 15% of women having a screening mammogram will be called back for additional imaging. Most of the time the findings of additional imaging will be benign.

Digital mammography is the newest form of breast imaging technology for screening. If available, it would be the preferred modality. It is especially beneficial for your patients who have dense breasts and who are at high risk for developing breast cancer.

Be specific and accurate in describing breast symptoms or problems when referring a patient for diagnostic imaging evaluation. Whenever possible, provide the patient with the necessary referrals so that all investigations can be carried out. This may require additional imaging studies and tests such as ultrasound, core biopsy, or both.

Breast ultrasound is beneficial as an adjunct imaging tool. It can define the extent of disease and differentiate solid masses (benign and malignant) from liquid-filled masses (cyts). Ultrasound is also is useful in evaluating causes of nipple discharge.

Breast MRI is highly sensitive (90%) but not very specific (70%) and is less helpful in evaluating ductal carcinoma in situ (DCIS). It is useful for assessing the following: multicentricity, multifocality, contralateral breast disease, axillary adenopathy, and assessing tumor response to neoadjuvant chemotherapy. It also is used for adjunct screening for patients with *BRCA1* and *BRCA2* mutations and women with greater than a 20% lifetime risk for breast cancer.

A percutaneous image-guided biopsy is recommended whenever possible. More than 90% of breast biopsies can be obtained in a minimally invasive manner without an incision or general anesthesia and still provide an accurate histopathologic diagnosis. However, they should be performed by a trained health care provider who specializes in these procedures.

What your patient needs to know:

Mammography remains the best method for early detection of breast cancer. Mammograms do not prevent breast cancer. Their use is intended to detect breast cancer at its earliest possible stage when it is easiest to treat and survival can be at its highest.

Women who are compliant with their annual screening mammograms have a higher probability of early diagnosis and survival according to studies that confirm that the use of screening mammograms has reduced breast cancer mortality by 30% to 60%.

Women should not panic if they are called back for additional imaging following a screening mammogram. Most will learn that the final outcome is benign.

Other forms of breast imaging, such as ultrasound, are not to be used as a substitute for screening mammograms. They are designed as adjunct imaging when needed and recommended.

The quality of the mammogram and its accuracy in identifying breast cancer correlate to some degree with the thoroughness the mammography technologist uses in ensuring that the breast is adequately compressed and that the maximal amount of breast tissue is captured on the image.

The radiologist who specializes in breast imaging usually makes the decision when additional imaging is needed, such as ultrasound or breast MRI.

Women should not attempt to read their own mammograms or ultrasound images.

They should go to a facility that is reputable and has shown interest in specializing in breast imaging.

If your patient has not received a copy of her results, she should call the facility and request them. All women and their ordering physicians are to receive written copies of their results.

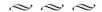

BENEFITS OF MAMMOGRAPHIC SCREENING

Randomized clinical trials performed over the last 40 years have shown a mortality reduction from breast cancer of approximately 30% in women offered screening mammography. It is very likely that the decrease in mortality attributable to screening mammography carried out in the community may be underestimated. There are estimates from Sweden that the mortality reduction from breast cancer is more on the order of 50% to 60%, attributed to early detection with mammography.[1, 2] Why the difference? Many factors could account for this:

▷ Marked improvement in mammographic technique and interpretation since the controlled clinical trials were carried out.

▷ Issues of compliance (in the U.S. studies, as many as 30% of patients invited to be in the study group did not show up for all their screening studies and have yet to be included in the final count).

▷ Number of screening rounds, length of follow-up, and length of screening intervals. All play a role in underestimating the benefits of mammography when compared to performance of annual mammography, every year, for a lifetime.

Although the benefits from screening mammography have repeatedly been contested since the early studies in the 1960s, the general consensus is that mammographic screening is beneficial in significantly reducing mortality related to breast cancer.

Since screening mammography was adopted on a widespread basis by physicians and women in the United States in the early 1990s, the mortality from breast cancer has dropped about 25% overall, mostly as a result of early detection with use of mammography.

WHO IS AT RISK FOR DEVELOPING BREAST CANCER?

More than 70% of breast cancers occur in women who have absolutely no identifiable risk factor other than being a woman and increasing in age. Breast cancer affects women predominantly after the age of 40. Less than 5% of breast cancers in developed countries occur in women younger than the age of 40. This may be different in other parts of the world where breast cancer incidence is not insignificant in younger women.

Family history of breast cancer in a first-degree relative or in multiple family members represents a significant added risk. In addition, 5% to 10% of breast cancers result from an inherited mutation, only few of which have been identified so far, such as the *BRCA1* and *BRCA2* genes. In such families the risk for developing breast cancer is high and may be on the order of 60% to 80%. Not infrequently in these families, the breast cancers develop at younger ages.

Hormonal factors such as early menarche and late menopause as well as late first pregnancy (after age 35) also affect breast cancer risk. Prolonged use of hormonal replacement therapy has been associated with an increased risk for breast cancer. The discontinuation of hormonal therapy in 2002 by many women following the discovery of this associated risk, for example, resulted in a lower incidence of breast cancer in 2003.

Women who have had prior breast biopsies that revealed proliferative changes are at higher risk for breast cancer; those with atypical cells found by pathology are at even higher risk.

Women who have developed cancer in one of their breasts are at higher risk for the development of another cancer in that same breast or in the contralateral breast.

RECOMMENDATIONS FOR MAMMOGRAPHIC SCREENING

It is recommended that all women older than age 40 have mammographic screening every year. For women older than 80, for whom the incidence of breast cancer starts to decrease, every other year may be adequate.

For women who have at least a first-degree relative with breast cancer, it is generally recommended that they start screening 5 years before the age at which the youngest family member was diagnosed with breast cancer. In families in which there are several members with breast cancer, including first-degree relatives, as well as in families with a genetic mutation, it is recommended that mammographic screening start 10 years before the age of diagnosis of the youngest family member with breast cancer.

It is clearly established that women whose cancer is localized to the breast have much better outcomes than those whose cancer has spread regionally to the lymph nodes or more distantly to metastatic sites. Even in patients with localized disease, the smaller the tumor, the better the outcome. A woman with a 1-cm breast malignancy has a much better prognosis than one with a 3-cm malignancy, with a 90% chance of being cured versus a 50% to 60% chance of being cured, respectively.

SCREENING MAMMOGRAPHY VERSUS DIAGNOSTIC MAMMOGRAPHY

When referring a patient for a mammogram, it is extremely important to decide whether the patient should be referred for a screening or diagnostic mammogram, as these are conducted differently.

A **screening mammogram** is an x-ray examination of the breasts of asymptomatic women in an attempt to detect abnormal lesions of the breasts when they are small and nonpalpable. Women complaining of vague bilateral breast pain qualify for a screening mammogram. Generally a screening mammogram is conducted without a physician on site. Rarely will the films be evaluated while the patient is at the facility, although the films are reviewed immediately for quality. The patients leave the facility and receive a letter in the mail a few days later informing them of the results of the examination. Five percent to 15% of patients may be called for additional imaging to evaluate an area of questionable or definite abnormality. Most of these patients will have a negative final outcome.

Conversely, a **diagnostic mammogram** is an examination used to evaluate a patient with a breast mass or breast masses as well as other breast signs or symptoms such as spontaneous nipple discharge, skin change, thickening, or nipple retraction. A diagnostic mammogram also includes women who are asked to return after the screening mammogram for further diagnostic imaging, women whose breast cancers were treated with breast conservation, and women with implants. The diagnostic examination is conducted in the presence of the radiologist who is monitoring the study, and the results are conveyed directly to the patient.

DIGITAL MAMMOGRAPHY VERSUS FILM SCREEN MAMMOGRAPHY

Digital mammography is the latest technology for x-ray imaging of the breasts. Results of the American College of Radiology (ACRIN) Digital Mammographic Imaging Screen Trial (DMIST) study published in 2005 comparing digital and film mammography have shown that digital mammography is more sensitive for the detection of breast cancer in women younger than 50 years, women with mammographically dense breasts, and premenopausal or perimenopausal women (www.cancer.gov/clinicaltrials/ACRIN_6652). In addition, digital technology allows the use of new applications that are not available for analog mammography, which include digital subtraction angiography, tomosynthesis (cross-sectional imaging), computer-aided detection (the equivalent of double reading), and electronic storage and transmission. The greatest impediment to the wide use of digital mammography is its cost. In 2006, less than 10% of the mammographic units in the United States were digital units. It will be several years before digital mammographic units will outnumber analog mammographic units.

There is no doubt that although mammography has its own limitations, whether digital or analog, we all depend on the technical quality of the mammogram and the expertise of the physician who is interpreting the study. Proper positioning and compression of the breasts, and proper density of the films are the technical components that will determine whether a cancer is detectable on the image. Since the introduction in 1992 of the Mammography Quality Standards Act (MQSA), there has been an improvement in the quality of mammograms. This is not, however, uniform in clinical practice. Similarly, the expertise of the interpreting physician is essential for the detection of the early and subtle cancers. Women are encouraged to get their mammograms at facilities that have demonstrated commitment to high-quality breast imaging and interpretation.

COMMUNICATIONS IN BREAST IMAGING

When referring a patient for a diagnostic evaluation, it is extremely important to be specific and accurate in describing the problem.

If the patient is referred for the evaluation of a focal abnormality in the breast such as a lump, one should describe the location of the abnormality by referring to the o'clock position on the breast and the number of centimeters from the nipple (actually measured with a ruler and not estimated).

If the patient is being referred for the evaluation of a discharge, one should note whether the discharge is spontaneous; unilateral or bilateral; from a single opening or multiple openings; and whether it is bloody, brownish, watery, mucoid, milky, or greenish.

BREAST ULTRASOUND

Breast ultrasound is an extremely important adjunct to mammographic imaging.[3] Indications for breast ultrasound include characterization of a palpable or mammographically detected mass—that is, whether it is a solid mass or a cyst. If the mass does not meet the criteria to be called a cyst, ultrasound aids in characterization by delineating the following: complex cyst; abscess; and benign-appearing, or malignant-appearing, or indeterminate-appearing mass.

Ultrasound is a necessary test for the evaluation of a definite lump or a question of a lump, irrespective of the age of the patient.

In the event of a mass being suspected or diagnosed to be a cancer, ultrasound is very helpful in delineating the extent of the disease within the breast immediately around the malignancy as well as evaluating the breast for multicentricity that is the presence of foci of cancer in the other quadrants of the breast. Breast ultrasound is also used to screen the contralateral breast for unsuspected malignancy (2% to 3% incidence).

In the presence of cancer, ultrasound evaluation of the axilla is carried out. If abnormal lymph nodes are detected, they can be biopsied percutaneously, usually by fine-needle aspiration (FNA).

Breast ultrasound is also used for the evaluation of nipple discharge when arising from a single opening (watery, mucoid, or bloody). In many instances an intraductal lesion may be seen.

Breast ultrasound is the primary modality for evaluating patients younger than age 30 who are referred for the evaluation of a lump. Mammography is rarely performed in patients younger than age 30.

Breast ultrasound screening is currently being evaluated.[4] Preliminary studies have shown that ultrasound screening will yield three cancers per 1000 screenings in high-risk individuals, nonpalpable and nonmammographically visible. More than 75% of these cancers have been stage 1. The problem with breast ultrasound is that it is operator dependent, physician intensive, and not reimbursed by insurance.

Finally, ultrasound is used to help perform image-guided percutaneous biopsy procedures.

BREAST MRI

Breast magnetic resonance imaging (MRI) has evolved as an extremely helpful tool for the evaluation of breast diseases.[5] It is extremely sensitive for the detection of invasive carcinoma of the breast, with sensitivity exceeding 90% and specificity of approximately 70%. It is less sensitive for ductal carcinoma in situ (DCIS). Current cancer-related indications for breast MRI include the following:

▷ Lesion characterization of proven or suspected cancer and delineation of extent of disease, including multifocality (within the same quadrant), multicentricity (cancer in other quadrants), and evaluation of the contralateral breast. Breast MRI may be considered if breast conservation surgery is very likely and there are concerns regarding the extent of the cancer.
▷ Axillary adenopathy proven to be caused by epithelial malignancy with a negative mammogram. MRI is helpful to identify the specific location of the primary tumor inside the breast.
▷ Grossly positive margins following lumpectomy with no preoperative MRI.
▷ Monitoring response to neoadjuvant chemotherapy for patients with locally advanced breast cancer.
▷ Suspicion of recurrent disease versus scar.

Although the sensitivity of MRI is high for invasive carcinoma, false negatives may be seen with DCIS and invasive lobular cancer, and, occasionally, with tubular carcinoma. In addition, there are a number of instances of false-positive MRI studies such as with fibrocystic change, proliferative changes, fibroadenoma, papilloma, and sclerosing adenosis.

Breast MRI screening is increasingly likely to be used for high-risk individuals, such as patients with a known mutation (i.e., *BRCA1* and *BRCA2*) and for individuals having multiple family members with a history of breast cancer without a mutation demonstrated or with lifetime risk greater than 20%. Breast MRI screening is not recommended for the general population of asymptomatic women.

If a suspicious lesion is detected on MRI that is not recognizable on the standard studies and does not correspond to anything visible on the mammogram, then a second-look ultrasound is recommended directed to the area of concern. If visible, the lesion may be biopsied under ultrasound guidance; if not, it may need to be biopsied under

MRI guidance. In addition, breast MRI is used for the evaluation of the augmented breast for implant integrity.

IMAGE-GUIDED BREAST BIOPSY

Percutaneous image-guided breast biopsies (ultrasound-guided, stereotactically guided, or MRI-guided biopsies) have almost totally replaced surgical excision for biopsy of a lesion from the breast.[6] The advantages are that the percutaneous image-guided biopsies are as accurate as surgical biopsies (with few exceptions), they are quick to perform, and they do not result in any scarring of the breasts. These procedures are very well tolerated and less expensive than surgical biopsy. If a diagnosis of benign disease is determined, then the lesion can be left alone and just simply monitored by periodic imaging. If the lesion is found to be malignant, then the patient can be spared a surgical biopsy and can go to a single, definitive surgical procedure.

If the lesion is visible under ultrasound, then it is easiest to biopsy under ultrasound guidance. If the lesion is not visible on ultrasound, which is most frequently the case with microcalcifications, then it would be biopsied under stereotactic guidance. If the lesion is detected only on MRI, even after a second-look ultrasound, then it may need to be biopsied using MRI guidance.

Whenever an image-guided biopsy of the breast is performed, the radiologist must make a statement whether the lesion was adequately and accurately sampled and whether the pathology and the imaging findings are concordant. If these are not concordant, then a recommendation to repeat the biopsy or resect the lesion should be made.

There are a few pathological findings on needle biopsy that are considered insufficient in that they may underestimate the disease process. These are atypical ductal hyperplasia, atypical lobular hyperplasia, and lobular carcinoma in situ. In those instances, surgical excision of the biopsy site is necessary. In more than 25% of cases with atypical cells, a more serious problem is discovered such as carcinoma in situ or invasive carcinoma. Any atypia on core biopsy should be followed by surgical excision.

The management of a diagnosis of papilloma on needle biopsy is controversial. There are significant instances in which surgical biopsy followed a diagnosis of papilloma and yielded, in addition, a diagnosis of DCIS. Some doctors prefer to resect all papillomas diagnosed by core biopsy; others are selective.

Finally, a diagnosis of a radial scar on core biopsy is considered insufficient, and surgical excision is warranted.

Most of the time an accurate diagnosis is made by needle biopsy indicating the presence of specific or nonspecific benign disease or of malignancy.

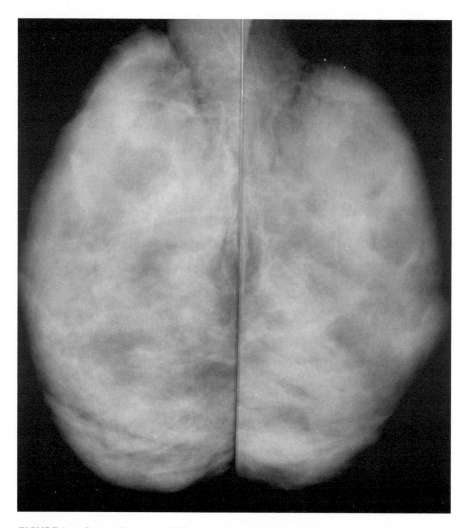

FIGURE 2.1 Dense Breasts. Oblique views of the breasts show dense tissues throughout. The sensitivity of mammography for the detection of masses is decreased in such breasts.

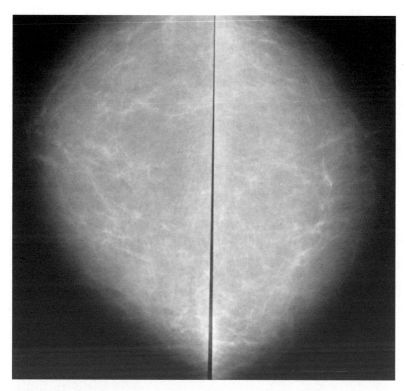

FIGURE 2.2 Fatty Breasts. Cranio-caudal views show the tissues to be predominantly fatty. The likelihood of detection of cancer in such a breast is very high even if the tumors are tiny, provided the involved area is included on the films.

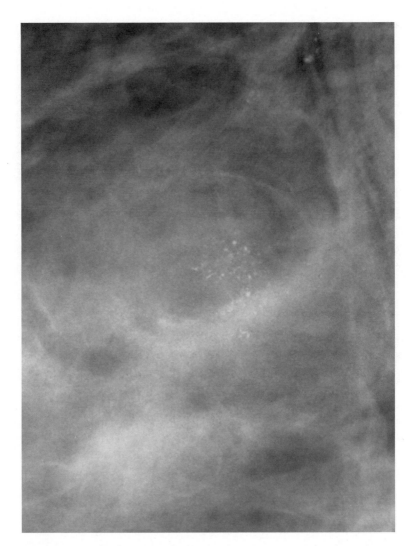

FIGURE 2.3 Tiny DCIS. Magnified view of a mammogram confirms the presence of a 5-mm suspicious cluster of microcalcifications in the upper left breast. Stereotactic biopsy yielded ductal carcinoma in situ. Chance of cure is 100%.

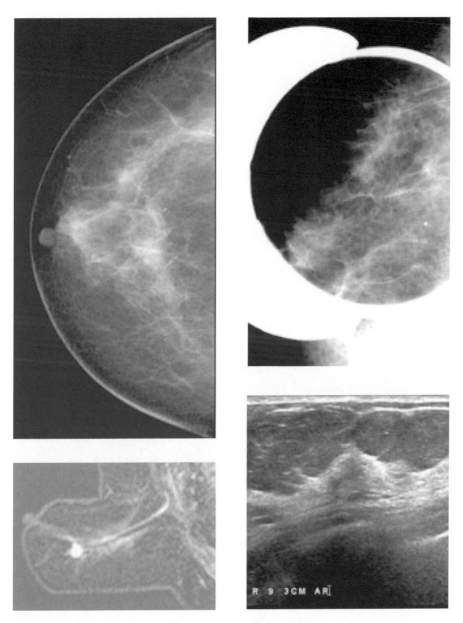

FIGURE 2.4 Small CA. Tiny, subtle 5-mm cancer confirmed on ultrasound in outer left breast. MRI confirms a single lesion that is circumscribed.

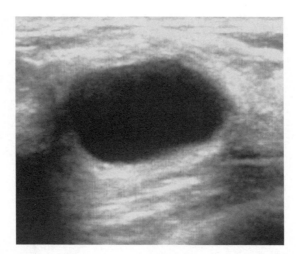

FIGURE 2.5 Cyst. Palpable mass in the breast evaluated by ultrasound shown to be a cyst.

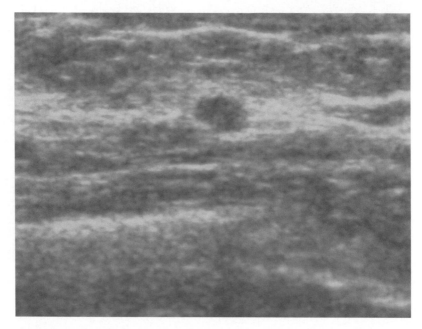

FIGURE 2.6 Small CA. A 45-year-old woman undergoing screening ultrasound because of a very strong family history for breast cancer: 4-mm cancer detected by ultrasound with a negative mammogram.

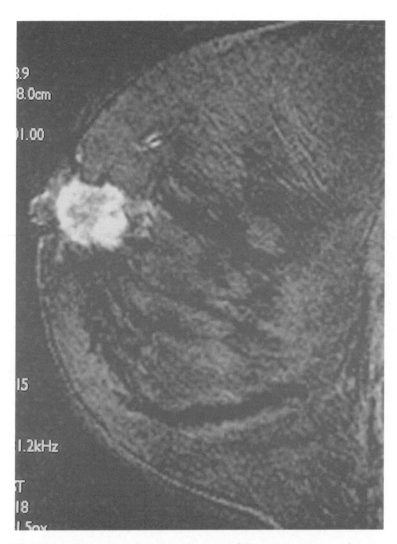

FIGURE 2.7 CA on MRI. Palpable suspicious fullness in a retro-areolar area of the left breast with a negative mammogram and vague findings on ultrasound. MRI clarifies the picture. Invasive carcinoma proven on core biopsy.

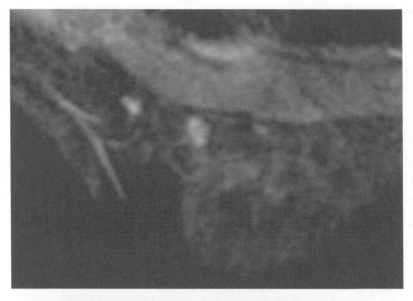

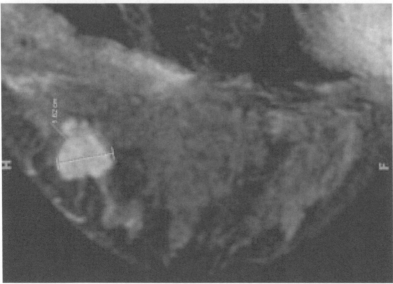

FIGURE 2.8 BIL CA on MRI. MRI performed for delineation of the extent of disease of proven carcinoma allows the detection of a contralateral cancer not suspected.

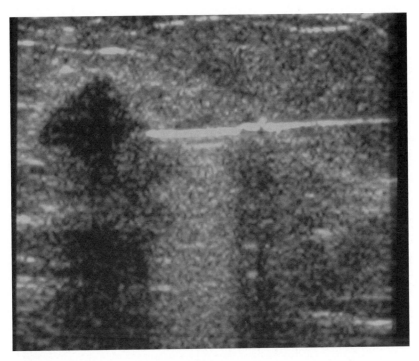

FIGURE 2.9 US Core. A core biopsy being performed under local anesthesia.

❧ Frequently Asked Questions

1. *My patient prefers to have ultrasound rather than mammogram for screening. Is this appropriate and adequate for evaluating and identifying early-stage breast cancer?*

   Mammography remains the gold standard for screening for breast cancer. Ultrasound is to be used as an adjunct tool for a breast evaluation. It is more appropriate for identifying and differentiating solid masses from cysts. Therefore, encourage your patient to continue to have annual mammograms for screening.

2. *My patient complains that mammograms hurt too much and therefore declines to get her screening annually. What does Johns Hopkins tell patients to promote compliance with screening?*

   We tell them that mammography is a screening test that takes only a few minutes. They are welcome to take over-the-counter analgesics prior to testing if their breasts are extremely sensitive. We reiterate the value of mammography in early detection of breast cancer. It also is helpful to explain why the compression is so tight—to be able to see through the breast tissue and provide an accurate reading of the images.

3. *If my patient is in her twenties and has a lump, is mammography the test that should be ordered for evaluation?*

   Breast tissue in young women is dense, and mammography may not be the ideal method of evaluation in these women. It is also more sensitive to radiation. It is more common to use ultrasound for evaluating women in this age group. To facilitate the diagnostic evaluation, be specific in your referral documentation as to the patient's symptoms/clinical findings and request that the radiologist in breast imaging determine the most appropriate method of diagnostic evaluation rather than specifying to the radiologist which tests you want done.

4. *I have routinely sent patients to a breast surgeon when I palpate a lump. Is this an appropriate referral process?*

   It is better to get a diagnosis before sending your patient to a surgeon. Sending your patient to a surgeon also increases her anxiety because she assumes she will need an operation. Direct her instead to a breast imaging facility for diagnostic evaluation, keeping in mind that more than 90% of biopsies can be done in breast imaging settings as core biopsies, without the need for an incision or general anesthesia. This technique is better for the patient and provides accurate information.

5. *Is digital mammography really superior to traditional analog film mammography?*

Yes, it is. When you look at the images side by side, you can really see the difference between them. The clarity of digital mammography is impressive, and it is especially helpful for women who are at high risk and for women with dense breasts. Although only a small percentage of breast imaging facilities currently have digital mammography, in the coming years more will adopt it, making it more readily available for your patients.

REFERENCES

1. Feig SA. Effect of screening mammography on population mortality from breast carcinoma. Cancer 2002;95:451–457.
2. Duffy SW, Tabar L, Chen H-H, et al. The impact of organized mammography service screening on breast carcinoma mortality in seven Swedish counties: A collaborative evaluation. Cancer 2002;95:458–469.
3. Mendelson EB. Problem solving ultrasound. Radiol Clin N Am 2004; 42:909–918.
4. Berg WA. Supplemental screening sonography in dense breasts. Radiol Clin N Am 2004;42:845–852.
5. Lee CH. Problem solving MR imaging of the breast. Radiol Clin N Am 2004;425:919–934.
6. Fajardo LL, Pisano ED, et al. Stereotactic and sonographic large core biopsy of a lone palpable breast lesion: Results of the Radiologic Diagnostic Oncology Group V study. Acad Radiol 2004;11:293–308.

Algorithm for Breast Pathology

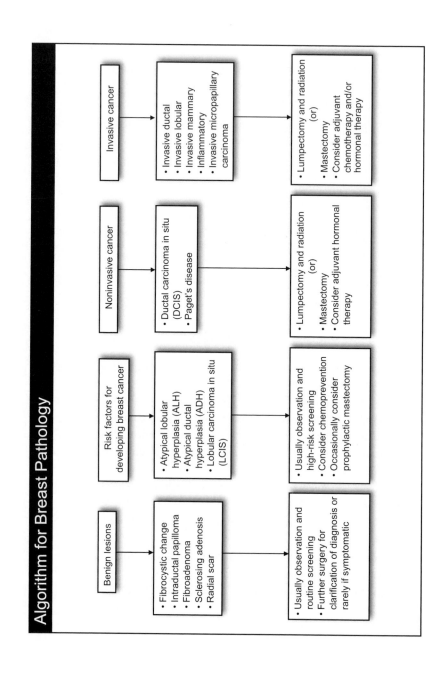

3

Understanding Breast Pathology

Pedram Argani, MD

What you need to know:

Benign lesions include fibrocystic changes, intraductal papillomas, fibroadenomas, sclerosing adenosis, and radial scars.

Risk factors that are found on a core biopsy and that warrant additional tissue sampling surgically of the area are atypical lobular hyperplasia (ALH—increases risk four- to fivefold), and atypical duct hyperplasia (ADH—increases risk four- to fivefold).

Ductal carcinoma in situ (DCIS) is a localized precursor to invasive breast cancer. It is also known as noninvasive breast cancer and stage 0 breast cancer. There are a variety of different types of DCIS.

Paget's disease refers to DCIS involving the nipple/areolar complex.

Lobular carcinoma in situ (LCIS) is a risk factor for breast cancer but is usually not treated like breast cancer, despite the confusion of its name containing "carcinoma." This is a point of confusion for some patients and warrants explanation.

There are a variety of types of invasive breast cancer, including ductal, lobular, mammary (which is a mixture of both ductal and lobular), and inflammatory. Invasive ductal is the most common type, followed by invasive lobular. Inflammatory breast cancer refers to carcinomas invading into and obstructing the lymphatics of the skin of the breast. It is a type at risk of missed diagnosis or delayed diagnosis, as its clinical presentation is different. It is aggressive and classified as stage 3 breast cancer based on the type and nature of breast cancer alone.

The five main prognostic factors for breast cancer are stage (based on tumor size, lymph node involvement, evidence of distant metastasis), grade, hormone receptors, proliferation index, and HER2/neu receptors.

A more unusual type of pathology is a phyllodes tumor. This is a neoplasm of the connective tissue of the breast (not the epithelium), which gives rise to carcinoma. Most such tumors are benign, but 10% will be malignant.

What your patient needs to know:

The accuracy of the pathologic diagnosis is critical to determining the stage and prognosis as well as the treatment plan.

There are different types of breast cancer. The most common is invasive ductal carcinoma, followed by invasive lobular carcinoma.

Thanks to early detection with mammography, more women are being diagnosed with DCIS—noninvasive breast cancer, stage 0 breast cancer.

Frozen sections are not to be done on breast tissue. The risk of inaccuracies is high and the tissue may be destroyed in the process. Frozen sections can be done on lymph nodes, however, such as the sentinel node.

Accurate pathologic evaluation usually takes several days and should not be rushed for the sake of trying to provide a fast answer to the patient. The website www.breastcancer.org offers a free brochure about how to explain pathology in terms for the layperson; this brochure can be obtained by mail or reviewed online.

INTRODUCTION

It is likely that you will be receiving a copy of your patient's pathology report from her needle core biopsy as well as her surgical procedure (lumpectomy or mastectomy). This chapter is intended to help clarify and review the significance of several of the terms that are found in those reports. The chapter is divided into a section that provides the definitions of common pathologic entities in the breast, followed by a section covering frequently asked breast pathology questions.

DEFINITIONS

Benign Lesions

FIBROCYSTIC CHANGES

Fibrocystic change is the most common cause of a breast mass in the United States. In addition, distended cysts may be painful, or epithelial hyperplasia may be associated with microcalcifications that are detected by mammogram. Fibrocystic change has three basic components: fibrosis, cysts, and usual duct epithelial hyperplasia. Simple fibrocystic changes, comprising fibrosis and cysts, pose no increased risk of breast cancer. Proliferative fibrocystic changes, which include usual duct epithelial hyperplasia, pose a minimal increased risk (1.5- to 2-fold) of subsequent breast cancer. This increased risk shows up in large population studies and, for the individual patient, is of little or no clinical significance. Patients with fibrocystic changes are typically given the usual follow-up.

INTRADUCTAL PAPILLOMA

Intraductal papilloma is a benign neoplasm that typically arises in the subareolar lactiferous ducts. Papillomas are composed of fibrovascular stalks lined by both benign secretory and myoepithelial cells. These may present as a subareolar mass or as bloody nipple discharge. When isolated and uncomplicated by other pathology, intraductal papillomas carry minimal increased risk of cancer. However, papillomas may be a fertile soil on which ductal carcinoma in situ (DCIS) or invasive ductal carcinoma may develop. Therefore, because lesions with the appearance of intraductal papilloma on a needle biopsy may be heterogeneous, complete but conservative excision is the usual treatment. Some patients have multiple small papillomas (micropapillomas) within the par-enchyma of the breast. These lesions are typically associated with proliferative fibrocystic changes.

FIBROADENOMA

Fibroadenomas are the most common benign neoplasms of the breast. These are typically well-circumscribed tumors that arise in young women 20 to 35 years of age. Microscopically, these are benign neoplasms of the intralobular fibrous stroma that induce proliferation of the entrapped terminal duct lobular unit epithelium. Simple fibroadenomas are associated with no increased risk of carcinoma. If the radiological findings are concordant, fibroadenomas identified on core needle biopsy may not require excision if the patient wishes to avoid surgery. Fibroadenomas in young patients (juvenile fibroadenomas) may be highly cellular and may recur. These should be distinguished from phyllodes tumors.

SCLEROSING ADENOSIS

Sclerosing adenosis is a benign increase in the number of glands (adenosis) accompanied by distorting myoepithelial cell proliferation, which distorts and narrows the lumens of the glands centrally (sclerosis). Sclerosing adenosis is a very common finding in benign breast biopsies and imparts minimal increased risk of breast cancer (approximately 1.5-fold, or the same risk implied by usual duct hyperplasia). Therefore, patients with these findings are generally given the usual follow-up.

RADIAL SCAR (COMPLEX SCLEROSING LESION)

Radial scars are benign lesions that mimic cancer mammographically and histologically. They have a stellate morphology with central sclerosis and elastosis that contains entrapped ducts, and a periphery that contains alternating cysts and ducts showing florid usual duct hyperplasia. Larger lesions (greater than 1 cm) often have superimposed papilloma or sclerosing adenosis, and are typically termed "complex sclerosing lesions."

Risk Factors for and Precursors of Invasive Carcinoma

ATYPICAL LOBULAR HYPERPLASIA (ALH)

ALH refers to cases in which cells morphologically indistinguishable from those of lobular carcinoma in situ (LCIS) are present within terminal duct lobular units, but the degree of distention of these units is insufficient to qualify for LCIS. As with LCIS, ALH is always an incidental finding diagnosed by the pathologist. This finding imparts a four- to fivefold increased risk of breast cancer that affects either breast. For more on this risk factor, see Chapter 15.

ATYPICAL DUCTAL HYPERPLASIA (ADH)

ADH refers to limited quantities of cells morphologically indistinguishable from those of low-grade DCIS. Essentially, the presence of a monotonous population of cells, which would otherwise qualify as low-grade DCIS but which measures less than 3 mm in greatest dimension, is the definition of ADH. When identified in excision biopsies, ADH is known to signify a four- to fivefold increased risk of breast cancer that is bilateral. When a needle core biopsy reveals ADH, conservative excision is generally indicated, because one may be sampling a small portion of a more extensive low-grade DCIS (the extent may not be evident on the fine-needle biopsy). When lesions with the morphology of ADH are present at a surgical excision margin, management is often difficult. If one is confident that the lesion has been completely excised, most physicians opt for no further surgery but close follow-up. However, if the ADH closely approaches the criteria for low-grade DCIS, and/or there is significant radiologic concern that there may be more lesional tissue remaining in the breast, many clinicians would recommend re-excision to obtain negative margins.

For more on this risk factor, see Chapter 7.

DUCTAL CARCINOMA IN SITU (DCIS)

DCIS refers to gland-forming carcinomas that are confined within the basement membrane of the terminal duct lobular units and larger ducts. Because these cells have not invaded into the surrounding stroma and do not have access to lymphatics or capillary vessels, these lesions cannot metastasize. Therefore, DCIS is a noninvasive cancer and is considered stage 0 (pTis). It originates from the terminal duct lobular units but tends to grow in large to medium-size ducts.

DCIS may have a variety of architectural patterns that make up the traditional classification of this lesion. These architectures are comedo, cribriform, micropapillary, solid, and papillary. However, in general, the nuclear grade of the lesion (graded on a scale of 1 to 3) is a more biologically and clinically significant distinguishing feature. Low-nuclear-grade (nuclear grade 1) DCIS is distinguished from ADH by the greater extent of the proliferation; most use 2 to 3 mm as the cutoff. No size cutoff is required to diagnose high-nuclear-grade (nuclear grade 3) DCIS.

DCIS is a localized precursor to invasive cancer; when untreated, the invasive cancers that follow almost always occur in the area of the DCIS. The risk is approximately 50% at 15 years for a low-grade DCIS and probably much greater for high-grade DCIS, although studies of the latter are limited. The treatment of DCIS involves complete excision, by either lumpectomy followed by radiation therapy, or mastectomy. If the DCIS expresses estrogen receptors, tamoxifen therapy can be offered as further prophylaxis against recurrence. Surgeons and radiation oncologists require a margin of at least 1 to 2 mm before declaring the excision to be adequate. Although DCIS should not have metastatic capacity, it is known that in patients with large, mass-forming, high-nuclear-grade DCIS, in approximately 1% to 2% of cases, disease may recur with metastatic disease. This likely reflects the presence of unsampled small foci of invasive high-grade carcinoma deep within these lesions, and the aggressive behavior of these high-grade invasive cancers.

PAGET'S DISEASE

Paget's disease refers to colonization of the epithelium of the nipple/areolar complex by the cells of DCIS, typically of the high nuclear grade, comedo type. Clinically Paget's disease presents with an eczematous rash involving the nipple. The demonstration of Paget's disease in a nipple biopsy signifies in almost all cases that a DCIS (at least) is present in the underlying breast. If a mass is detected in the breast on clinical examination, it is more likely that an invasive carcinoma has already evolved from the DCIS. This is in contrast to the situation with Paget's disease of the vulva or anus, where an underlying visceral organ carcinoma is less frequently identified. The important clinical point is that lesions that resemble eczema involving the nipple should be considered suspicious for Paget's disease until proven otherwise. The presence of Paget's disease does not impart any diminished prognosis when evaluating the underlying DCIS or invasive carcinoma, although it typically necessitates excision of the nipple.

LOBULAR CARCINOMA IN SITU (LCIS)

LCIS does not form a distinct mass, and usually does not calcify; it is usually an incidental finding by the pathologist in a biopsy performed for another lesion (such as fibroadenoma or fibrocystic changes). LCIS is characterized by filling, distention, and distortion of the terminal duct lobular units by small, dyscohesive uniform cells with round nuclei and often vacuolated cytoplasm. Gland formation is absent. LCIS cells (and the cells of invasive lobular carcinoma) lack expression of the

E-cadherin protein, which correlates with their dyscohesive nature. Unlike with DCIS, the risk of subsequent cancer posed by LCIS is bilateral. For many years it has been assumed that the risk is equal in both breasts, so treatment for LCIS has ranged from close observation to bilateral prophylactic mastectomy. More recent data suggest that the risk is skewed toward the ipsilateral breast (approximately 3:1), although not nearly as ipsilaterally skewed as the risk for DCIS. Tamoxifen prophylaxis is also considered as a potential preventive measure for patients who have LCIS. For more on this risk factor, see Chapter 14.

Cancers

INVASIVE DUCTAL CARCINOMA

Invasive ductal carcinoma refers to a cancer of the epithelial lining cells (secretory cells) that has extended outside the terminal duct lobular units and large ducts and into the mammary stroma. The majority (more than 80%) of breast cancers are invasive ductal carcinomas. The malignant secretory cells form glands to some degree; well-differentiated (Elston grade 1) cancers have bland nuclei, have few mitoses, and form glands throughout, whereas poorly differentiated (Elston grade 3) carcinomas tend to have variably sized nuclei, have abundant mitoses, and grow in a sheetlike pattern. The five favorable subtypes of invasive breast carcinoma (tubular, cribriform, colloid, adenoid cystic, and medullary) are considered subtypes of invasive ductal carcinoma.

INVASIVE LOBULAR CARCINOMA

Invasive lobular carcinoma is characterized by small, round, uniform cells that invade in linear, concentric patterns. The cells of invasive lobular carcinoma are cytologically identical to those of LCIS. Compared to invasive ductal carcinomas, invasive lobular carcinomas are more often bilateral, are harder to define grossly and therefore occult clinically, and metastasize preferentially to different sites. For example, invasive lobular carcinoma preferentially metastasizes to the gastrointestinal tract viscera, serosa of the abdomen, and meninges. Most invasive lobular carcinomas prove to be Elston grade 2 (moderately differentiated). However, when matched grade for grade, there is no prognostic significance to distinguishing invasive ductal carcinoma and invasive lobular carcinoma.

INVASIVE MAMMARY CARCINOMA

Invasive mammary carcinoma refers to an invasive carcinoma with features of both invasive ductal carcinoma and invasive lobular carcinoma. The prognosis is not affected by having mixed ductal and lobular differentiation.

INFLAMMATORY CARCINOMA

Inflammatory carcinoma refers to an invasive carcinoma that has invaded into and obstructed the lymphatics of the skin of the breast, producing an orange-peel-like appearance to the skin of the breast. Patients with this type of carcinoma typically have systemic disease and, therefore, a poor prognosis. The diagnosis of inflammatory carcinoma is based on clinical findings with pathologic correlates. Histologically, the presence of carcinoma within lymphatics of the skin alone, in the absence of clinical findings, does not equate with inflammatory carcinoma.

INVASIVE MICROPAPILLARY CARCINOMA

Invasive micropapillary carcinoma refers to an invasive carcinoma that histologically resembles metastatic serous carcinoma of the ovary. In fact, it is not uncommon for pathologists to have trouble distinguishing between the two without immunohistochemical staining. The main significance of invasive micropapillary carcinomas is that these tumors tend to present at an advanced stage. However, when stage is accounted for, prognosis is no different from that for typical invasive ductal carcinoma.

Other

PHYLLODES TUMOR

A phyllodes tumor is considered to be the more aggressive counterpart of a fibroadenoma. Once again, this is a biphasic tumor in which the neoplastic stroma induces proliferation of the entrapped benign epithelium. The cellular proliferating stroma typically undermines the epithelium to give leaflike protrusions. Phyllodes tumors are distinguished from fibroadenoma histologically by the prominent leaflike pattern and the increased stromal cellularity, atypia, and mitotic activity. Although these lesions were previously known as "cystosarcoma phyllodes," the fact is that most of these (more than 90%) are benign, with potential only for local recurrence.

Phyllodes tumors can be subdivided into three types: benign, low-grade malignant/borderline, and high-grade malignant. The benign phyllodes tumor has potential for local recurrence when incompletely excised, but no metastatic capacity. The low-grade malignant/borderline phyllodes tumor has significant potential for aggressive local recurrence, but virtually no metastatic capacity. The high-grade malignant phyllodes tumor behaves essentially as a sarcoma; 25% will metastasize in a hematogenous fashion. It should be emphasized that the majority of phyllodes tumors are local control problems and have minimal risk of metastasis. The optimal treatment is complete excision of these tumors.

∿ Frequently Asked Questions

1. What are the main prognostic factors in breast cancer?

The five main prognostic factors are stage (determined by tumor size, lymph node status, and distant metastases—TNM), grade proliferation index, estrogen and progesterone receptors, HER2/neu amplification, and proliferation index. Of these, stage is by far the most important prognostic factor.

2. How is tumor size determined?

The size of a breast cancer may be determined grossly in the pathology lab when the pathologist cuts the specimen and measures the tumor with a ruler. However, sometimes what appears as a grossly evident mass may not be invasive carcinoma but rather DCIS or scar. In cases such as this, the measurement of the tumor is best made on the basis of microscopic measurements rather than gross measurements. That is, the pathologist examines the tumor under the microscope and measures the greatest extent of invasive carcinoma on the slides. The prognosis—and, therefore, the stage of the tumor—is based on the invasive component (the size of the invasive carcinoma, not the DCIS). This measurement often requires correlation of gross and microscopic findings.

3. How is the node stage determined?

Traditionally the axillary lymph nodes were assessed by a formal axillary lymph node dissection, which typically yielded approximately ten lymph nodes. Now, the axilla can be assessed by examining the sentinel node, which is the first node in the axilla to which dye or radioactive tracer injected into the breast drains. If the sentinel lymph node has metastatic carcinoma, a formal complete axillary dissection is typically performed. However, if the sentinel node is free of carcinoma, the rest of the axilla will very likely not have carcinoma, and, therefore, an axillary dissection can be safely omitted.

Because resection of the sentinel node yields a smaller amount of tissue than a full axillary dissection, it can be examined carefully to look for small foci of metastatic carcinoma. In some laboratories, immunohistochemistry for cytokeratin is used to detect small metastases. However, the nodal involvement is classified according to the size of the metastatic tumor deposits, not how they are detected. For example, small clusters of tumor cells measuring less than 0.2 mm, without evidence of mitoses or stromal reaction, are considered isolated tumor cells (ITCs), which are considered pN0 (node-negative for clinical purposes). Tumor deposits of smaller than 2 mm but larger than 0.2 mm are considered micrometastases (pN1mi). Metastases larger than 2 mm are considered macro-metastases (pN1). The number of lymph nodes with micrometastasis or macrometastasis determines stage. Tumors with one to three positive nodes are considered pN1, four to nine positive nodes are considered pN2, and ten or more positive nodes are considered pN3.

4. How can the sentinel node be assessed intraoperatively?

Many surgeons ask pathologists to assess the sentinel node intraoperatively so that if it is positive (i.e., contains metastasis), an axillary dissection can be performed while the patient is still under anesthesia. Frozen section is the traditional method of examining tissue intraoperatively; however, frozen section may deplete and cause severe artifacts within fatty axillary sentinel nodes, thereby compromising their interpretation. Hence, instead of frozen sections, some pathologists prefer cytologic smears (Touch Preps) of the sentinel node. Either way, it is expected that there will be a small false-negative rate, because the entire node cannot be examined at the time of frozen section. Occasionally small deposits of tumor will appear on the permanent sections that are prepared and interpreted a few days later. Whether a formal axillary dissection should subsequently be performed depends on the individual clinical scenario for that patient. Sometimes axillary radiation can be substituted for complete axillary dissection.

5. *How are estrogen and progesterone receptors determined on an invasive breast carcinoma?*

In the "old days," estrogen and progesterone receptors were determined using a biochemical method (such as charcoal binding assays), which required frozen tissue. Hence, breast cancers were sent for frozen section examination, partly so that sufficient tissue could be procured for this analysis at the time of operation. This methodology has several major flaws, the main ones being that it wastes tumor that otherwise could be examined histologically; it requires frozen sections, which distorts tissue such that diagnosis may be impossible; and it may not be accurate (because contaminating normal breast tissue within a specimen could give a false-positive hormone receptor result). Currently almost all laboratories use an immunohistochemical assay for estrogen and progesterone receptors. Several of these methods have been calibrated to clinical outcome (i.e., response to antiestrogen therapy) and, therefore, are clinically validated tests. In general, the assessment of staining for estrogen and progesterone receptors is based on the proportion of the cells that stain and the intensity of staining. This is sometimes known as the "Allred score," named after the pathologist (D. Craig Allred) who created this scoring system.[1] In general, **any positive staining is potentially significant,** and as little as 1% labeling of tumor cells may predict some benefit from relatively nontoxic antiestrogen therapy. Therefore, it is important that the slides be examined thoroughly to identify any estrogen- or progesterone-receptor staining, and that the internal controls on the slides be labeled appropriately to assure that the assay is working (normal breast epithelium is usually positive with these assays, so it is a good internal control). A good policy is for the laboratory to report the percentage of invasive carcinoma cells that stain and the intensity of staining.

Allred Score = Proportion Score + Intensity Score

Proportion Score

0: no staining

1: <1% staining

2: 1% to 10% staining

3: 10% to 33% staining

4: 33% to 66% staining

5: >66% staining

Intensity Score

0: none

1: weak

2: intermediate

3: strong

The Allred score has a possible range of 0 to 8.

6. *How is HER-2/neu overexpression determined?*

The HER2/neu oncogene, present on chromosome 17, is amplified in approximately 15% of invasive breast carcinomas. Amplification of this tyrosine kinase results in overexpression of the HER2/neu protein. In normal breast epithelium, HER2/neu protein is not detectable immunohistochemically, but it does become detectable in the subset of tumors in which the gene is amplified.

The traditional method for detecting HER2/neu overexpression is immunohistochemistry. Scoring is generally on a scale of 0 to 3+. In general, tumors that show no staining or minimal staining (0 or 1+ score, respectively) virtually never have gene amplification, whereas tumors that show strong, complete membranous staining (3+ score) almost always have HER2/neu gene amplification. Tumors that show equivocal staining (2+ score) may or may not have amplification; most laboratories send these cases for fluorescence in situ hybridization (FISH) assessment of HER2/neu gene amplification. In general, HER2/neu gene amplification studies are thought to better predict response to Herceptin (trastuzamab) therapy (although this is not completely established) and may be less affected by variables such as fixation, which can dramatically alter HER2/neu immunohistochemical staining. There is, therefore, a push toward greater utilization of FISH in breast cancer cases. Tumors with HER2/neu amplification usually have a ratio of HER2/neu probe to centromere probe of 5 or more (the normal ratio is 1). Tumors with a ratio of less than 1.8 are considered nonamplified, whereas those with a ratio in the range of 1.8 to 2.2 are in the "borderline amplification" category. The clinical significance of borderline amplification remains to be determined.

7. How is grade determined?

The typical grading system used in invasive breast carcinoma is the Elston grading system. In this system, invasive carcinomas are scored on the basis of tubule formation, nuclear atypia, and mitoses.

▷ Tubule formation is scored as follows: greater than 75% tubules, 1 point; 10% to 75% tubules, 2 points; less than 10% tubules, 3 points.

▷ Nuclear pleomorphism is scored as follows: minimal pleomorphism, 1 point; moderate pleomorphism, 2 points; marked pleomorphism, 3 points.

▷ Mitotic figures are scored per surface area. Using a standard ocular high-power objective with a diameter of 0.59 mm, the scoring is as follows: fewer than 9 mitoses per 10 high-power fields, 1 point; 10 to 19 mitoses per 10 high-power fields, 2 points; 20 mitoses or more per 10 high-power fields, 3 points.

The scores for each of these components are then added to give a final Elston grade for the tumor. Tumors with Elston scores of 3 to 5 are Elston grade 1, those with scores of 6 to 7 are Elston grade 2, and those with scores of 8 to 9 are Elston grade 3.

8. What are the favorable subtypes of invasive breast cancer?

The five favorable subtypes are

▷ Invasive tubular carcinoma

▷ Invasive colloid carcinoma

▷ Invasive cribriform carcinoma

▷ Invasive adenoid cystic carcinoma

▷ Invasive medullary carcinoma

Invasive tubular carcinoma is typically an incidental finding, often picked up on mammogram. It is composed of very well-formed tubules, which are sometimes difficult to distinguish from the benign ducts of the breast.

Invasive colloid carcinoma typically forms a smooth, rounded mass in an elderly patient, and hence can be mistaken for a fibroadenoma clinically. Histologically this tumor is defined by bland tumor cells floating in a sea of extracellular mucin.

Invasive cribriform carcinoma is a low-nuclear-grade tumor that resembles cribriform DCIS of the breast, except that it has an invasive growth pattern.

Invasive adenoid cystic carcinoma of the breast is histologically identical to its aggressive namesake in the salivary gland. Despite the fact that this tumor is typically nonimmunoreactive for estrogen and progesterone receptors, it is associated with an excellent prognosis.

Invasive medullary carcinoma is a controversial topic; most studies claim that it has a better prognosis than the typical invasive ductal carcinoma with prominent lymphocytes, but not all studies do. This is likely because pathologists disagree about the criteria for a true, pure medullary carcinoma. The key features are a circumscribed border, a syncytial growth pattern of tumor cells, and a dense lymphoplasmacytic infiltrate. Patients with BRCA1 mutations frequently develop tumors with medullary features.

9. *What are the "S-phase fraction (SPF)" and the Ki-67 index?*

These criteria are basically measurements of how rapidly the tumor cells are dividing or proliferating. The S-phase is the stage in the cell cycle where DNA is synthesized; it occurs just before a cell divides. The S-phase fraction is measured by flow cytometry. It is easiest to perform on fresh tissue, but can be applied to formalin-fixed tissue blocks, although the results may be suboptimal. Another downside of this technique is that there are really no interlaboratory standards for a normal SPF; different laboratories establish their own ranges.

At Johns Hopkins, we use the Ki-67 immunohistochemical stain to measure proliferation. We favor this technique because it allows us to assess proliferation only of the tumor cells, because we see the tissue on the slide that stains for Ki-67. In our laboratory, the mean Ki-67 index for an invasive breast cancer is 20%, less than 10% is considered a low Ki-67 index, and greater than 30% is considered high.

10. Which prognostic factors can be determined accurately on a needle core biopsy?

Clinicians frequently wish to determine the patient's stage prior to therapeutic intervention so that options such as preoperative chemotherapy can be considered. Unfortunately, not all prognostic factors can be determined accurately by noninvasive needle core biopsies of the breast and fine-needle aspiration of axillary lymph nodes.

In terms of stage, tumor size is difficult to determine on a core biopsy. The largest area of invasive carcinoma seen on a core biopsy is usually approximately 1 cm. However, when a core biopsy reveals invasive ductal carcinoma, one cannot assume that a clinically or radiologically defined 3-cm mass is all invasive carcinoma, because scarring and DCIS may account for a significant proportion of the mass. Therefore, clinical and radiologic size determinations may be inaccurate. Axillary lymph nodes may be staged by fine-needle aspiration. A positive result (metastatic carcinoma identified by fine-needle aspiration) is reliable. However, a negative fine-needle aspiration result is not always reassuring; approximately 10% of cases will prove to be false negatives (i.e., there was carcinoma present in the lymph nodes, but it was not sampled by the needle aspiration). Distant metastases can be accurately diagnosed by needle biopsy, provided that the biopsy is large enough to allow for confirmatory immunohistochemical staining that proves the carcinoma originated in the breast.

In terms of tumor grade, high-grade invasive cancers on needle core biopsy almost always prove to be high-grade invasive cancers on excision. However, lesions that appear to be low-grade invasive carcinomas on needle core biopsy may prove to be high grade on excision. Therefore, only a high Elston grade identified on needle biopsy is accurate.

Immunohistochemical stains for hormone receptors (estrogen and progesterone receptors) and HER2/neu are generally accurate when determined on needle core biopsy. Proliferation index is often inaccurate, because the core biopsy may sample the hypoxic center of the tumor and miss the highly proliferative leading edge of the tumor at its periphery. One cannot accurately determine whether a tumor is of special favorable type histology on needle core biopsy, because this requires complete examination of the entire lesion histologically.

To summarize, one can accurately determine that a patient has a node-positive high-grade invasive cancer on core biopsy, and accurately determine the hormone receptor and HER2/neu status. In the absence of documented node-positive disease, prognostic factors determined on needle core biopsy may be inaccurate.

11. What kind of prognostic information can be determined after preoperative chemotherapy has been given?

Locally advanced tumors are frequently treated by preoperative chemotherapy. This allows a potentially unresectable lesion to be resected. Some clinicians, particularly in the setting of a research trial, offer patients preoperative chemotherapy for operable breast cancers. It is important to recognize that many of the key prognostic factors in breast cancer are lost after preoperative chemotherapy. Tumor size may be impossible to determine accurately due to asymmetric tumor shrinkage. Lymph nodes may show areas of scarring and fibrosis after chemotherapy; in this setting, it may be difficult to determine whether there was metastatic carcinoma present that was destroyed by effective chemotherapy, or whether the scarring and fibrosis represent a nonspecific reaction in a lymph node that never harbored a metastasis. The significance of Elston grade is unknown after chemotherapy, because chemotherapy artificially changes the factors (nuclear atypia, tubule formation, and mitotic count) that are used to determine Elston grade. Proliferation index is of unproven value in the postchemotherapy setting. Hormone receptors and HER2/neu are generally consistent between the preoperative biopsy and the postchemotherapy specimen. Special type histology is of no known significance after chemotherapy. Margins may be particularly difficult to determine after chemotherapy, because the tumor may adopt a bland appearance, which may be difficult to distinguish from macrophages. There is evidence that higher rates of local recurrence are seen in women who require chemotherapy to undergo breast conservation. Hence, particularly in node-negative patients with breast cancer, preoperative chemotherapy results in a significant loss of prognostic information.

After chemotherapy, pathologists attempt to assess the efficacy of the treatment. Because the preoperative size of the tumor cannot be accurately determined, the contribution of chemotherapy is difficult to assess. A pathologic complete response (pCR) is defined as no invasive carcinoma present in the breast. The general consensus is that patients with viable metastatic carcinoma in the axilla should be excluded from the pCR category, although not all studies (such as NSABP B-27) have used this criterion. The presence of in situ carcinoma is compatible with the pathologic complete response. Although some studies suggest that the pathologic complete response is a favorable prognostic factor, this is not true of all studies. Indeed, in NSABP B-27, the addition of docetaxel doubled the pCR rate, but resulted in no significant difference in overall or disease-free survival. It is clear that in patients who have pathologic complete responses, disease may recur and they may eventually die from breast cancer. Hence, the significance of a pCR remains to be proven.

12. *How are margins defined?*

After a breast specimen (lumpectomy or mastectomy) is delivered to pathology, the edges of the specimen are inked so that the pathologist can determine whether the carcinoma extends to these edges. These edges are the margins of the specimens. If carcinoma (DCIS or invasive carcinoma) involves these margins or is very close to them, further surgery to obtain negative margins (free of carcinoma) is indicated. How far should carcinoma be from the margins before the margin is considered negative? This criterion varies between institutions and depends on the characteristics of the tumor; however, most accept a clearance of 1 to 2 mm or more to be adequate.

For a lumpectomy, the specimen can be thought of as a cube, so there are six margins to be assessed (superior, inferior, medial, lateral, anterior, and posterior). If the specimen is oriented by the surgeon as to how it lies in the patient, the pathologist can differentially ink each margin with a different color (red, blue, black, green, yellow, and orange) so that the pathologist can accurately determine which margins are involved. Given this information, the surgeon may not need to re-excise all of the margins on re-operation when only a few of them are positive; instead, he or she may opt to obtain extra tissue only in these specific involved areas. Many surgeons now submit additional margins (cavity margins) at the time of a lumpectomy, to supersede the margins of the specimen. These extra shave margins are taken after the lumpectomy has been removed, and they represent the true margins of the specimen. This method results in a significant decrease in positive margins, likely due to the elimination of artifactually positive specimen margins.[2]

In a mastectomy, the key margins are the deep margin (which faces the chest wall) and the superficial margin, which faces the skin. These are also inked differentially such that they can be distinguished. Positive margins in this setting may or may not trigger postmastectomy radiation therapy.

13. Should frozen sections be done on breast biopsies?

The answer is almost always "No!" Frozen sections used to be done to establish the diagnosis of invasive carcinoma, so that the surgeon could proceed to mastectomy while the patient was under anesthesia, and the pathologist could select fresh tissue for biochemical estrogen- and progesterone-receptor analysis. However, both of these reasons are now outdated. First, radiologically guided needle core biopsy now allows the diagnosis of invasive carcinoma to be established without the need for open biopsy. Options for therapy (i.e., lumpectomy plus radiation versus mastectomy) can, therefore, be evaluated before definitive surgery. Second, we now can test for estrogen and progesterone receptors on fixed tissue using immunohistochemistry, so fresh tissue is not needed for this purpose. Hence, the former benefits of frozen section are no longer relevant.

Frozen sections do have significant disadvantages. First, frozen sections are difficult to interpret, and are more likely to be misinterpreted by a pathologist than are the usual permanent slides. For example, benign inflammatory cells can be difficult to distinguish from infiltrating lobular carcinoma on frozen sections. Second, the process of freezing tissue introduces considerable artifacts that can make the lesion impossible to diagnose. For example, it is well known that frozen section artifact can make it impossible to distinguish a benign papilloma from a papillary carcinoma, because it is hard to appreciate the myoepithelial cells that accompany a papilloma, which are absent in a papillary carcinoma. In addition, immunohistochemical stains may not always be easily interpreted in tissue that has been frozen. Finally, small lesions, such as are detected mammographically, may be depleted or even completely lost in the process of rapidly trimming the tissue in a frozen section cryostat. Such lesions are better handled carefully under standard processing (parenthetically, a similar argument can be made against performing frozen sections on sentinel lymph nodes). Hence, we generally do not perform frozen sections on breast specimens at Johns Hopkins.

14. *What is a good format for planning the care of a patient with breast disease?*

Multidisciplinary tumor boards are particularly useful for discussion of the optimal therapy for patients with breast disease. In this format, the clinical presentation and exam findings can be presented by the surgeon, radiology reviewed by the radiologist, biopsy pathology reviewed by the pathologist, and decisions regarding potential adjuvant therapy discussed by the medical oncologist (chemotherapist) and radiation oncologist (radiation therapist). This multidisciplinary approach ensures that all members of the team are fully aware of the significance of the patient's lesions, the risks imposed by these lesions, and the potential benefits and harms imposed by proposed therapies.

REFERENCES

1. Harvey JM, Clark GM, Osborne CK, Allred DC. Estrogen receptor status by immunohistochemistry is superior to the ligand-binding assay for predicting response to adjuvant endocrine therapy in breast cancer. J. Clin Oncol 1999;17:1474–1481.
2. Cao D, Lin C, Woo S-H, et al. Separate cavity margin sampling at the time of initial breast lumpectomy significantly reduces the need for re-excisions. Am J Surg Path 2005;29:1625–1632.

Algorithm for Treatment of Noninvasive Breast Cancer

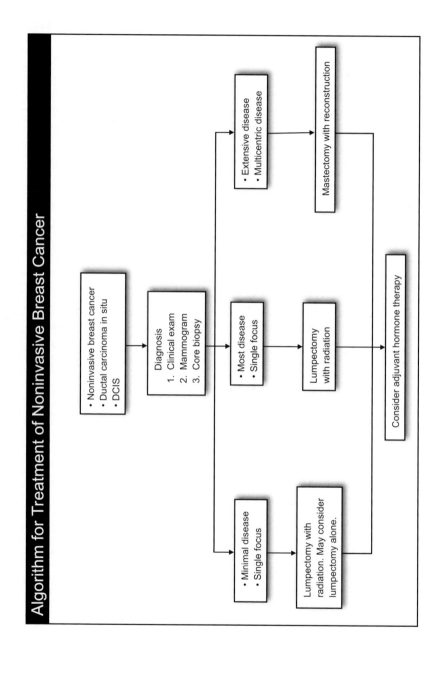

Algorithm for Treatment of Invasive Breast Cancer

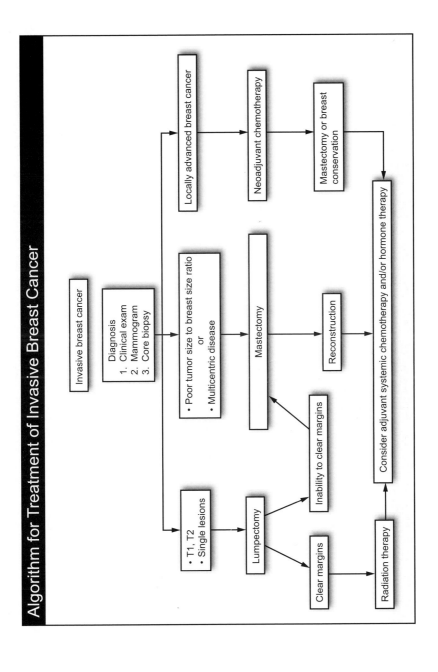

Algorithm for Treatment of the Axilla in Breast Cancer

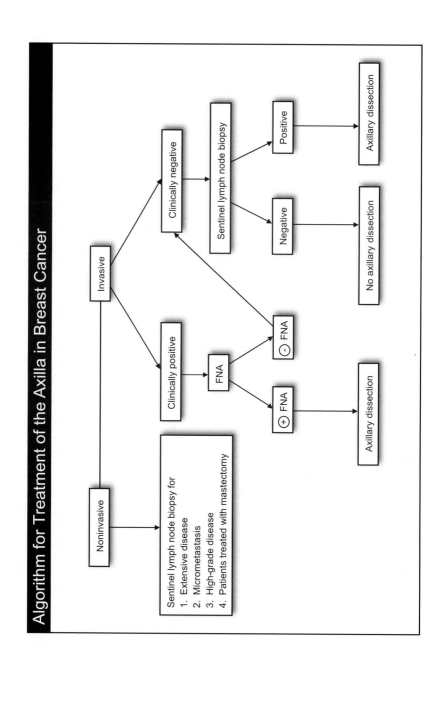

chapter

4

Breast Cancer: Surgical Options and Management

Theodore N. Tsangaris, MD

What you need to know:

Core biopsy is preferred to excisional biopsy.

Lumpectomy and radiation provide equal disease-free survival and overall survival rates when compared to mastectomy.

Extensive metastatic work-ups are inappropriate in most situations.

All patients, regardless of stage and surgical procedure, should see a medical oncologist and a radiation oncologist.

What your patient needs to know:

A core biopsy does not introduce cancer into the system and does not cause metastatic spread. In fact, a core biopsy is the safest way to biopsy and preserve all future treatment options.

Mastectomy should be considered for large tumor size-to-breast size ratio and for patients with multicentric disease. All others should consider breast conservation.

Mastectomy is not a surgical substitute for chemotherapy or other systemic therapy.

For women who do require mastectomy, immediate reconstruction is preferable.

INTRODUCTION

For the health care provider, the increasing incidence of breast cancer coupled with the increased sophistication of treatment for these patients can be extremely challenging. Therefore, knowing how to appropriately introduce the patient into the multidisciplinary team for the treatment of breast cancer is very important.

PREOPERATIVE EVALUATION

Traditionally the surgeon was most often the first contact for the woman identified with a breast problem. Most primary health care providers are more than happy to quickly transfer the patient and her breast problem to the surgeon. However, a good clinical examination by the individual referring that patient and a diagnostic mammogram are not only appropriate but will facilitate any further work-up. It is important to realize that the first thing a surgeon will do is order a diagnostic mammogram. Therefore, it makes sense to do this on initial presentation. Breast radiologists are now very proactive and often during a diagnostic mammogram will start with initial images, engage in further work-up of the problem with additional images, and biopsy the lesion when appropriate, thereby making the diagnosis even before the surgeon sees that patient. Often the diagnosis of a simple cyst or other benign finding can help the patient avoid seeing the surgeon altogether. Therefore, we would strongly encourage primary health care providers to refer their patients to competent Breast Centers for a diagnostic mammographic work-up when presented with a patient with a breast problem.

When a biopsy is warranted, core biopsy and fine-needle aspiration (FNA) have essentially replaced the excisional biopsy. At Johns Hopkins we prefer core biopsy because of the histologic information it provides. Not only are these biopsy options accurate, but they are minimally invasive and help maintain the integrity of the breast. An untimely excisional biopsy is often detrimental to the patient. It can make obtaining clear margins difficult, impede the sentinel lymph node procedure, or blemish an otherwise outstanding skin-sparing mastectomy with reconstruction. At our institution we will perform excisional biopsy only when core biopsy is equivocal or discordant and the additional tissue will clarify the diagnosis. An incisional biopsy should almost never be performed.

Once cancer is diagnosed it is very important to convey a sense of purpose but not panic to the patient. There is no emergency here. Given the natural history of most breast cancers (a 1-cm invasive cancer has been present for 3 to 5 years), a rush to treatment is inappropriate and actually harmful. There are too many options for the patient to quickly decide upon, and a second opinion may be necessary. Furthermore, one should attempt to dispel the myth that biopsy encourages the tumor to grow. The "larger" lump is probably secondary to trauma [yes, even FNA can cause a hematoma] and that axillary node is very likely reactive to the biopsy. One to two weeks is a reasonable time from biopsy to definitive surgical treatment. In cases where mastectomy and reconstruction are required, a 4- to 6-week delay may be necessary. Some patients may just need time to weigh their options.

WORK-UP

In cases where cancer is diagnosed, an extensive systemic work-up is not appropriate. For most early-stage breast cancer patients, a good history and clinical examination along with bilateral mammograms are adequate. Chest x-ray and blood work are actually used for preoperative clearance. Should a patient present with evidence of locally advanced disease, have pathologically positive lymph nodes, or raise suspicion through clinical symptoms at initial presentation, a metastatic work-up is indicated. In summary, the initial presentation of a breast problem warrants the following:

1. History and physical examination
2. Diagnostic mammogram
3. FNA or core biopsy (when indicated)
4. Surgical consultation (when indicated)

BREAST CANCER

Simply stated, breast cancer is either invasive or noninvasive. Noninvasive cancer is essentially a local disease, whereas invasive cancer is both a local and potentially a systemic disease. Although both are often treated locally with identical surgical approaches, we discuss these diseases separately.

INVASIVE BREAST CANCER

Finding the correct approach for treating invasive breast cancer is less controversial than the approach to noninvasive disease. However, arriving at the most appropriate surgical treatment for invasive disease can still be emotionally and intellectually challenging for all involved.

The systemic treatment for invasive cancer is discussed in subsequent chapters. Suffice it to say that all patients with invasive breast cancer at Johns Hopkins see a medical oncologist after surgery, regardless of the stage.

Most patients with early-stage breast cancer should be considered for breast conservation (lumpectomy and radiation therapy). Relative contraindications to breast conservation include (1) large breast cancers relative to a small breast size, (2) inability to receive radiation therapy, and (3) multicentric disease. The National Surgical Adjuvant Breast and Bowel Project (NSABP)-B06 trial and numerous other trials since the 1970s support without reservation the equality of breast conservation and mastectomy. Disease-free survival and overall survival rates are identical for these options. It is inaccurate and inappropriate to prejudice a patient toward "more aggressive" surgery as a means of achieving better survival results.

SURGICAL CONSIDERATIONS

For single lesions of appropriate tumor size–breast size ratio, lumpectomy should be the procedure of choice. The basic principles of lumpectomy are as follows. First, the incision should reflect the skin tension lines of the breast, usually a curvilinear incision. The incisions should be placed directly over the tumor and tunneling should be avoided. Accurate placement of the incision facilitates radiation therapy and follow-up. It also provides the best cosmetic outcome in most situations. Excising the tumor and obtaining adequate margins around the cancer while preserving cosmetic integrity are the primary goals of the surgeon.

We define a 2-mm to 3-mm microscopic margin as a free margin. It is very important that the specimen be handled carefully so that its integrity and its orientation are maintained. The pathologist uses colored ink to designate the margins. Positive or close margins can, therefore, be more accurately and efficiently dealt with. Before closure of the lumpectomy incision, microclips are placed to delineate the tumor cavity radiographically for the radiation oncologist and the mammographer.

The technique of mastectomy has not changed significantly, except that skin sparing when possible should be considered. For those patients who need or prefer mastectomy, strong consideration should be given for immediate reconstruction. Reconstruction has become highly sophisticated and provides outstanding cosmetic results. Skin-sparing mastectomies set up the plastic surgeon with a canvas to achieve truly remarkable artistic results. The types of reconstruction options available will be described in later chapters. However, it should be understood that the type of reconstruction should be based on the cosmetic and physiologic needs of the patient. The type of cancer should have little impact on the decision of the plastic surgeon except in those situations of locally advanced disease in which postmastectomy radiation will be utilized. Delayed permanent reconstruction, in which a tissue expander is initially used, should be considered in these cases.

Regardless of the surgical treatment chosen for the breast, axillary sampling of the ipsilateral axilla should be performed. The standard of care today is the sentinel lymph node (SLN) biopsy for a clinically negative axilla. In principle, the SLN biopsy identifies the axillary lymph node most likely to have tumor if tumor has metastasized to the axilla. Three methods have survived early trials: one uses a vital blue dye injected into the breast, one uses a radioactive isotope, and the third uses both techniques. The surgeon's familiarity, experience, and confidence with a chosen SLN biopsy technique are more important than the specific method is employed. It is our practice to perform an intraoperative histologic examination of the sentinel lymph node. If the node is positive, then axillary dissection is performed at that operative sitting. This approach in our institution is very successful, with only a 5% to 6% discordance rate between frozen section and permanent section. Our sentinel lymph nodes are analyzed with standard hematoxylin and eosin (H&E) staining.

A formal axillary dissection should be performed for a positive sentinel lymph node or clinically suspicious axilla. A level 1 dissection would seem justified in most cases, as there is a diminishing return of lymph nodes obtained and an increase in morbidity when the surgeon moves into level 2 and level 3.

NEOADJUVANT THERAPY

For patients with locally advanced disease, consideration should be given to primary or neoadjuvant chemotherapy, and surgery should be delayed. Neoadjuvant chemotherapy has gained increased popularity and use in an effort to make the surgical procedure easier. Often mastectomy patients are converted to lumpectomy patients after completion of treatment. Although across-the-board survival benefits have yet to be realized, neoadjuvant therapy provides important prognostic information and will be vital as a research tool to gain insight into the biologic behavior of breast cancer. During the neoadjuvant period it is important that the surgeon see the patient sometime during the course of treatment. At Johns Hopkins we try to make that first visit halfway through the treatment. It is during this visit that progress can be assessed and preliminary surgical plans made. After completion of chemotherapy and a final follow-up examination, mammograms and other tests are obtained, and surgical plans are finalized with the patient.

NONINVASIVE BREAST CANCER

Over the years the incidence of noninvasive breast cancer (DCIS, or ductal carcinoma in situ) has increased. The increased incidence of DCIS clearly parallels the increased use of screening mammography. Given that DCIS is essentially a local disease, which is highly curable with surgery alone, the surgeon must recognize that the treatment for noninvasive breast cancer will vary from individual to individual. This disease can present the surgeon and the patient with several emotional and intellectual challenges. A balanced approach to treatment is important. Maintaining cosmetic integrity of the breast while reducing the risk of local recurrence can be difficult. Generally the same criteria used for invasive disease are applicable to noninvasive disease. Lumpectomy with radiation is preferred for most women.

There have been both large prospective trials and smaller retrospective trials that have supported breast conservation. The NSABP and other groups have shown in large prospective trials that lumpectomy and radiation are equivalent to mastectomy in terms of their overall and disease-free survival rates. Other investigators have suggested that lumpectomy alone is sufficient for most patients with noninvasive breast cancer. The Van Nuys pathologic classification and Van Nuys prognostic index are the cornerstones of this treatment option. At Johns Hopkins most of our noninvasive patients receive radiation after lumpectomy.

As with invasive disease, mastectomy is appropriate for large areas of DCIS relative to breast size, or multicentric disease. Mastectomy with immediate reconstruction should also be considered in these situations.

Sentinel lymph node biopsy for DCIS is reserved for patients with extensive disease, micrometastases, high-grade lesions, or patients requiring mastectomy.

ADJUVANT THERAPIES

All women with invasive and noninvasive breast cancer should give consideration to systemic adjuvant therapy. Such therapy includes chemotherapy and hormonal therapy for invasive cancer and hormonal therapy for noninvasive disease. Treatment should be based on the patient's age, general condition, and tumor prognostic and predictive factors. Adjuvant therapy is discussed in greater detail elsewhere.

Radiation therapy after lumpectomy should be considered standard care for invasive and most noninvasive disease. Standard therapy consists of whole-breast radiation with a boost to the tumor bed covering approximately 6 weeks. New treatments such as partial-breast radiation are promising and are being provided at Johns Hopkins and other institutions in a protocol setting.

The indications for postmastectomy radiation are less clear and somewhat controversial. Recent studies have suggested that patients with tumors of a certain size, histologic characteristics, or positive lymph nodes may benefit from postmastectomy radiation. A recent overview of the postmastectomy radiation data suggests its use for even one positive lymph node. Currently at Johns Hopkins, however, the widespread use of postmastectomy radiation is closely scrutinized.

CONCLUSION

The surgeon's role in the care of the breast cancer patient is no longer limited to the operating room. The Halstead radical mastectomy has given way to a more sophisticated total approach, and the surgeon must manage his or her patient within a multidisciplinary approach to the breast disease. This certainly explains the development and proliferation of the dedicated Breast Center and breast specialist.

⌒ Frequently Asked Questions

1. *I have been diagnosed with a worrisome finding on mammogram and I want it taken out ASAP. Will the needles cause my cancer to spread?*

   It is better to have the lesions diagnosed with a tissue sample taken with a core biopsy first. It is an old wives' tale that needle biopsy will cause spread of breast cancer.

2. *Shouldn't I have a bone scan, CT scan, and PET scan to see if my breast cancer has spread?*

   The current recommendations suggest that a good history and physical examination and using the tumor staging and prognostic characteristics are the most appropriate way to screen for metastatic disease.

3. *If I have a mastectomy, will I ever have to worry about breast cancer again?*

   Mastectomy is preferred for large breast cancers and multicentric breast cancers in establishing local control. It does not improve overall survival or alter subsequent systemic therapy or follow-up.

4. *Is it safe to have immediate reconstruction after a mastectomy?*

   It is absolutely safe to have immediate reconstruction after mastectomy. Occasionally the final reconstruction is delayed after placement of an expander while the patient is completing her systemic and local radiation, if necessary.

FURTHER READING

Fisher B, Anderson S, Bryant J, et al. Twenty-year follow up of a randomized trial comparing total mastectomy, lumpectomy and lumpectomy plus irradiation for the treatment of invasive breast cancer. N Engl J Med 2002;347:1233–1241.

Fisher B, Dignam J, Wolmark N, et al. Tamoxifen in treatment of intraductal breast cancer: National Surgical Breast and Bowel Project B-24 randomized controlled trial. Lancet 1999;353:1993–2000.

Algorithm for Breast Reconstruction

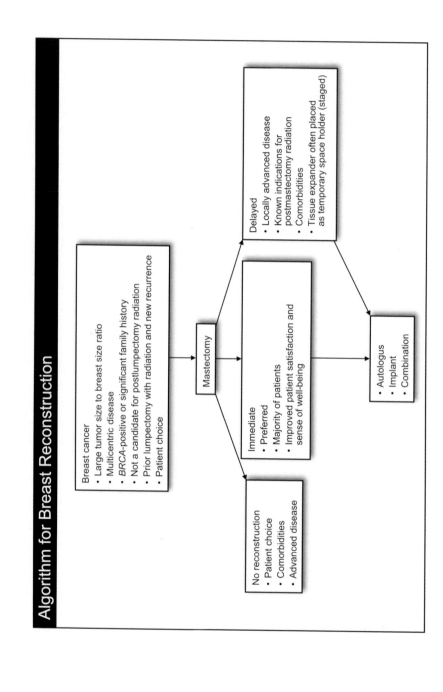

Breast cancer
- Large tumor size to breast size ratio
- Multicentric disease
- *BRCA*-positive or significant family history
- Not a candidate for postlumpectomy radiation
- Prior lumpectomy with radiation and new recurrence
- Patient choice

Mastectomy

No reconstruction
- Patient choice
- Comorbidities
- Advanced disease

Immediate
- Preferred
- Majority of patients
- Improved patient satisfaction and sense of well-being

Delayed
- Locally advanced disease
- Known indications for postmastectomy radiation
- Comorbidities
- Tissue expander often placed as temporary space holder (staged)

- Autologus
- Implant
- Combination

5

Breast Reconstruction

Navin K. Singh, MD, MBA, FACS
Gedge D. Rosson, MD

What you need to know:

Breast reconstruction for women who have had a diagnosis of breast cancer is a covered expense by insurance companies thanks to the Women's Health and Cancer Rights Act (WHCRA) of 1998, which mandates coverage. This coverage includes alteration of the contralateral breast to ensure symmetry.

The majority of women needing or choosing mastectomy will be good candidates for some form of breast reconstruction. Women can choose to have reconstruction done immediately at the time of mastectomy or as a delayed procedure done some time after mastectomy.

Today there are a variety of methods for reconstructing the breast, including the use of implants (saline or silicone), or some form of tissue transfer—pedicled transverse rectus abdominus myocutaneous (TRAM) flap, free TRAM flap, deep inferior epigastric perforator (DIEP) flap, latissimus dorsi flap, or superior gluteal artery perforator (S-GAP) flap.

Reconstruction is usually a multistage process. The finale will be nipple reconstruction and areola tattooing.

Patients should be nicotine-free for at least 6 weeks prior to reconstructive surgery. This includes having completed transition from smoking to patch or gum to nothing at time of surgery. This is due to the risk of vasoconstricton that leads to tissue ischemia.

Diabetics are at higher risk for having small blood vessels and increased risk of poor wound healing. Coronary artery disease also affects blood flow and the success of reconstruction.

Women having DIEP flap reconstruction have less risk of hernia later in life than those having TRAM flap reconstruction. This is a key reason that DIEP flap is preferred.[1,2] In addition, there are no lifting restrictions for patients having DIEP flap once the postoperative healing is complete. Problems with bulge are also less frequent. However, the vessel used for the anastomosis is commonly the internal mammary (IM) artery, which is the same vessel that cardiac surgeons use for coronary revascularization in treating patients with coronary artery disease (CAD). Arterial conduits, such as IM artery–left internal mammary artery (LIMA) or radial artery grafts, have been shown to have a greater patency rate than saphenous vein grafts. Cardiac surgeons usually prefer these vessels, so in the event your patient needs coronary artery bypass grafting (CABG), the patient and her cardiac surgeon should review the operative report from her flap reconstruction to see which vessels were used. CAD may be more likely in women having radiation to the chest wall and, in particular, if their breast cancer was in the left breast.

A three-dimensional (3-D) computed tomography (CT) angiogram is sometimes done by the plastic surgeon in advance of the flap surgery to help identify the status of the vascular perforators in the abdominal muscle, and to preselect the area that appears to have the best vessels.

What your patient needs to know:

Women having mastectomy surgery have the right to receive reconstruction. Sometimes women do not discuss this issue with their surgeons because their attention is focused on survival and a faster recovery. Reconstruction should be discussed in depth with the patient, and all the various types of reconstruction reviewed to help her select the one that is best for her.

Women who opt not to have reconstruction done at time of mastectomy surgery, or for medical reasons cannot, have not burned their bridge by declining, however. Reconstruction can be done later—even years later.

Before 1998, breast reconstruction, even for someone with a diagnosis of breast cancer, was considered cosmetic surgery and was not covered by insurance. Since 1998, all forms of reconstruction have been covered, and are covered for the lifetime of the patient, including if she changes insurance companies, opts for a different type of reconstruction later (i.e., choosing to do implant first and then electing DIEP flap later), and/or has body size changes that result in asymmetry (i.e., weight gain that results in the natural breast being larger than the implant side).

Women should look at breast reconstruction as a short-term investment for a long-term gain.

> Doing reconstruction at the time of mastectomy does not negatively affect proceeding with additional adjuvant therapy such as chemotherapy, and does not delay its start date.[3]

~ ~ ~

INTRODUCTION

The American College of Surgeons estimates that women's lifetime risk for breast cancer may be as high as 1 in 7. Approximately 75,000 women had breast reconstruction last year, which represents an approximately 150% increase from 1992. This increase in reconstruction is due partly to greater access to care, to more patient education, and to the passage of the WHCRA of 1998, which mandates insurance coverage for reconstruction and alteration of the contralateral breast for symmetry.

Most of our patients seek immediate breast reconstruction when they are contemplating a mastectomy. We feel privileged to provide this option to patients, and often it makes the decision to undergo a mastectomy more palatable when several good options for reconstruction are available. If their tumor biology and location are suitable, patients should also consider lumpectomy plus radiation as one of their choices, and pursue an informed discussion with their plastic surgeon and radiation oncologist (Figure 5.1). Women with a very strong family history of breast cancer (with or without *BRCA* mutation) may desire a bilateral mastectomy to reduce future risk and thus bilateral reconstruction.

Nonetheless, occasionally a woman will have too many medical comorbidities to undergo reconstruction, such that prolonged anesthesia or invasive surgery may prove a greater hazard than any potential benefit. A handful of women are advised to delay reconstruction until they have both physically and mentally recuperated from the mastectomy. Studies have shown that women who have "grieved the loss of a breast" are much more enthusiastic about their reconstruction when one is achieved, as compared to women who had immediate reconstruction. Several clinicians feel that a woman who goes to sleep with one breast and wakes up with a substitute breast after a

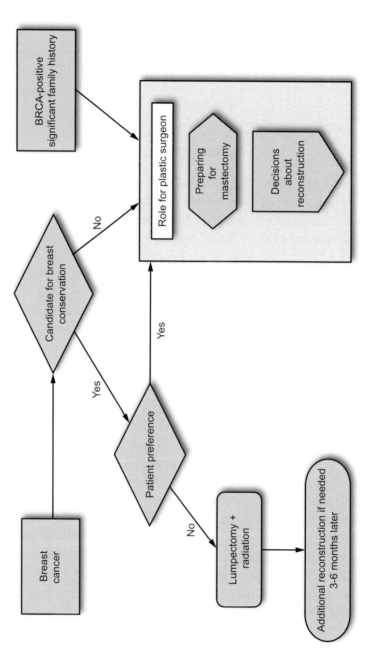

FIGURE 5.1 Deciding Between Lumpectomy Versus Mastectomy

combined oncologic–plastic procedure for immediate breast reconstruction will not be as accepting or as tolerant of the limitations.

Rarer still are the women who are good candidates, whose tumor is not advanced, but who nevertheless do not want to pursue breast reconstruction. Typically these are very active and athletic women who are trying to not let the cancer take away any more of their time than is absolutely necessary. In our 24/7 culture, physicians and nurses need to empower their patients to give themselves permission to heal and to take the time to pursue the best options available, not just the most expedient. I tell my patients, "Time is not of the essence. You are!"

Ultimately the role of the physician is that of a waiter: I tell patients what's on the menu and advise them of the physical costs/risks associated with each item, and let them choose what they want to eat.[4] An experienced surgeon, like a good waiter, can also tell the patient what the chef recommends—and allow his or her experience to benefit the novice.

Once she has decided on mastectomy, the patient can choose whether she wants immediate breast reconstruction or delayed breast reconstruction (Figure 5.2).

Reconstructive options are depicted in Figure 5.3.

The reconstructive options are as follows, in increasing order of complexity:

1. No reconstruction
2. Two-stage implant reconstruction
   a. First stage—expander
   b. Second stage—saline or silicone implant
3. Single-stage implant reconstruction
   a. Using tissue replacement matrix
4. Pedicled transverse rectus abdominis musculocutaneous flap (TRAM)
5. Pedicled back tissue
   a. Latissimus dorsi flap
   b. Thoracodorsal artery perforator flap (TDAP)
6. Microsurgical free flaps
   a. Free TRAM
   b. Free TUTG (transverse upper thigh Gracilis)
   c. Free DIEP (deep inferior epigastric artery perforator)
   d. Free SGAP (superior gluteal artery perforator)
   e. Free IGAP (inferior gluteal artery perforator)

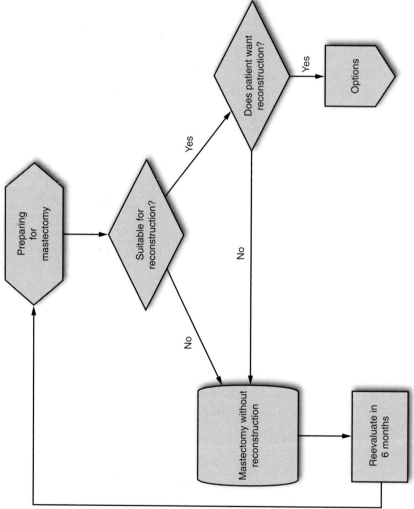

FIGURE 5.2 Evaluation for Immediate Reconstruction

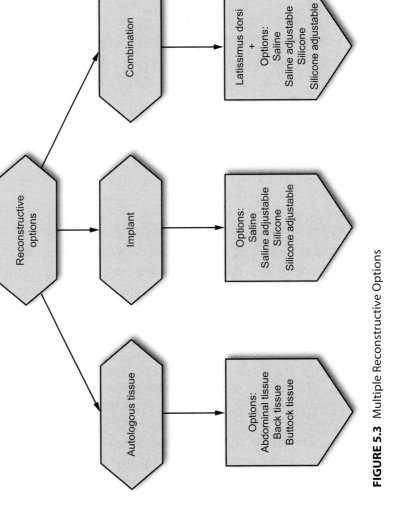

FIGURE 5.3 Multiple Reconstructive Options

PREOPERATIVE PLANNING

Our center is using 3-D perforator mapping of the abdomen to identify vessels (Figure 5.5). These data are currently preliminary but suggest a role for increased accuracy and decreased operating room time by preoperatively mapping the perforator and knowing its location.

Patients should undergo teaching via face-to-face time with the surgeon and/or designee such as a mid-level practitioner [e.g., nurse practitioner (NP), physician's assistant (PA)]. Brochures, videos, and other teaching tools can be used in addition to one-on-one time with the health care provider for educating the patient. We prefer to have the patient's husband or significant other participate in the process.

Patients should have preoperative teaching regarding the details of the procedures and options from both the surgical oncologist and plastic surgery perspectives. We also like our patients to meet with the physical therapist preoperatively as well as to learn gentle range-of-motion and core-strengthening exercises.

Some centers require preoperative autologous blood donation (PABD) to prepare for flap surgery. At our center, the need to transfuse for flap surgery arises so infrequently that it does not warrant PABD. Patients are educated nonetheless about the risks and benefits of potential blood transfusion, including the possibility of transfusion reaction and infection.

OPERATIVE PROCEDURES

Implant-based reconstruction at the time of mastectomy usually requires an overnight hospitalization, whereas autologous tissue reconstruction (Figure 5.4) requires approximately 3 to 4 days in the hospital. Similarly, the overall time to recuperate and return to work is longer for autologous tissue reconstruction.

Centers with higher volumes tend to have better outcomes because surgeons, nursing teams, and postoperative care become very standardized and consistent. When experience is concentrated in a few hands, outcomes improve. Further, a plastic surgeon who routinely devotes a significant portion of his or her practice to breast reconstruction is important for the center—as that individual will have

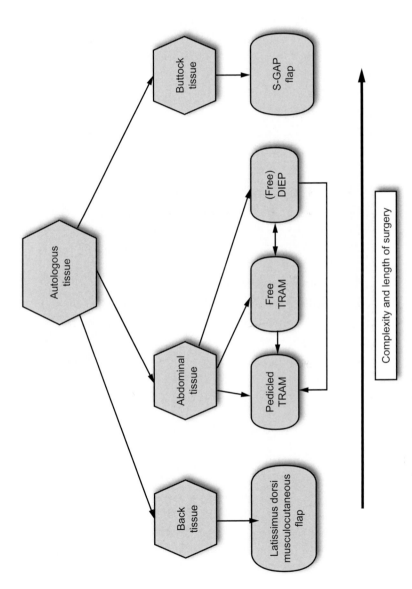

FIGURE 5.4 Autologous Tissue Options

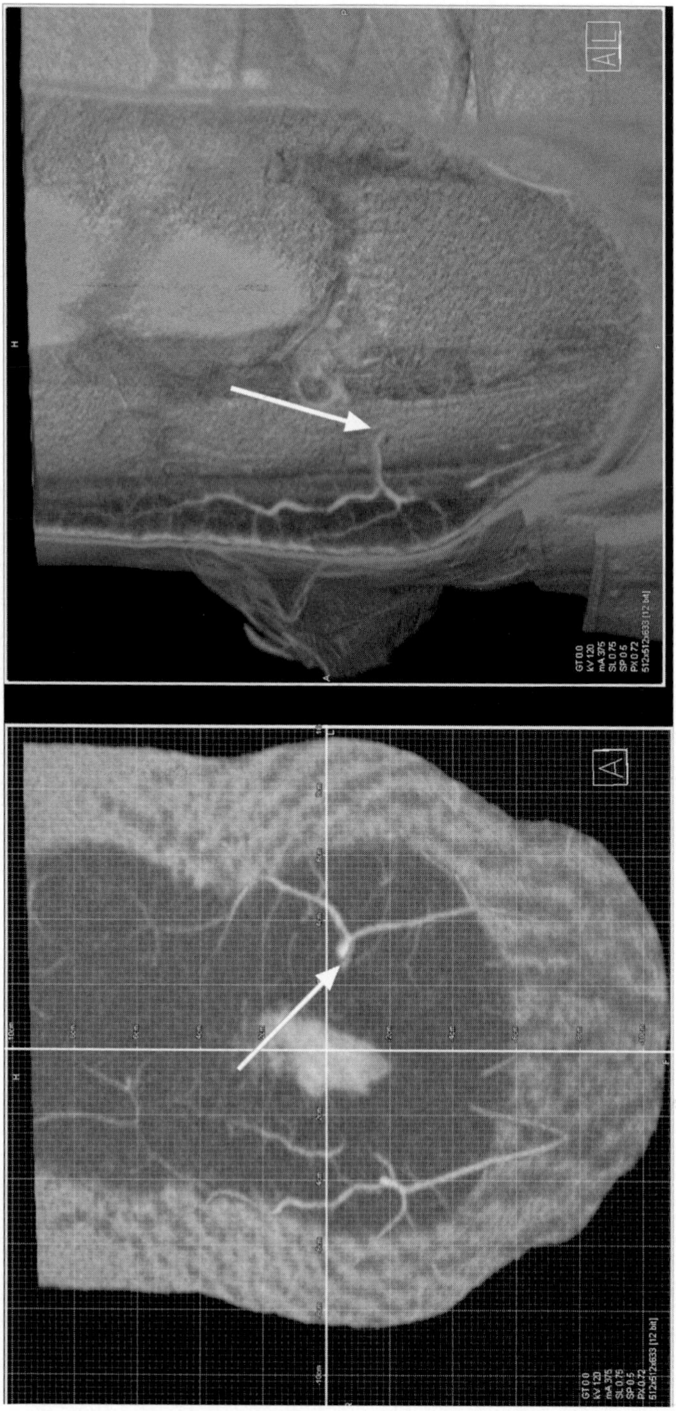

FIGURE 5.5 Mapping Abdominal Perforators in Preparation for DIEP Flap Surgery

great familiarity with the protocols and indications, a track record of teamwork with the oncologic surgeons, and the infrastructure to support a patient.

Postoperative care includes the following measures:

1. Showers allowed in 2 days.
2. No heavy lifting for 4 to 6 weeks. This allows the donor sites to heal without risk of hernia formation [in the case of TRAM flaps and DIEP flaps (Figure 5.6)] or disruption of the various layers and distortion of the ultimate aesthetic result of the reconstruction. The body continues to increase collagen content of a healing wound for up to 6 weeks. At that stage, collagen turnover and remodeling take over.
3. Antibiotics are used perioperatively, and rarely do they need to be continued after discharge from the hospital.
4. Gentle physical therapy exercises to encourage range of motion.

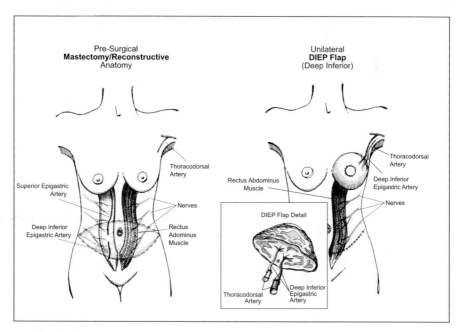

FIGURE 5.6 (left) Presurgical mastectomy/reconstructive anatomy. (right) Unilateral DIEP flap.

A PICTURE IS WORTH A THOUSAND WORDS

Implant-Based Reconstruction

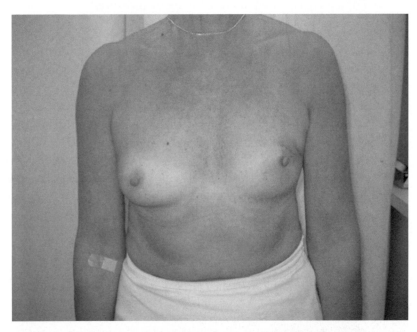

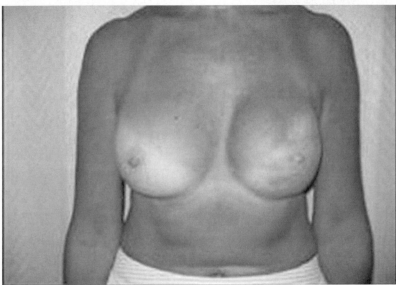

FIGURE 5.7   (top) Preoperative; (bottom) Left implant reconstruction with right augmentation for symmetry.

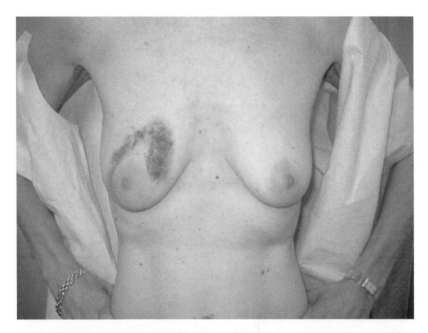

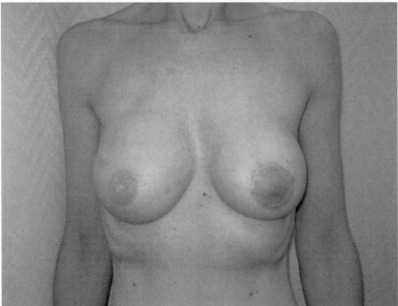

FIGURE 5.7(continued) (top) Preoperative; (bottom) Right implant reconstruction with left augmentation for symmetry.

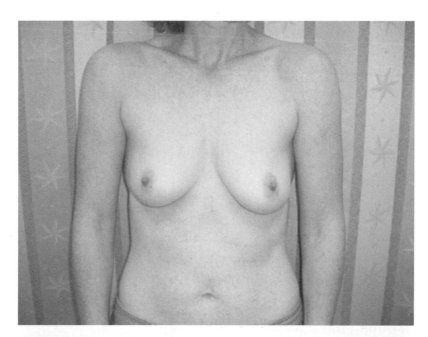

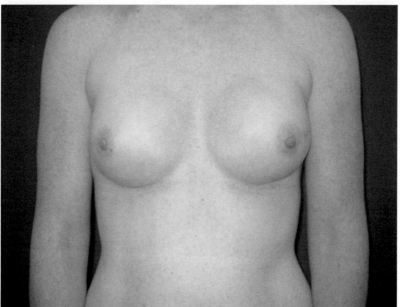

FIGURE 5.8 Nipple-sparing mastectomy with one-stage implant reconstruction with Alloderm used. (top) preoperative, (bottom) postoperative

Latissimus Dorsi Flap and TDAP Flap Reconstruction

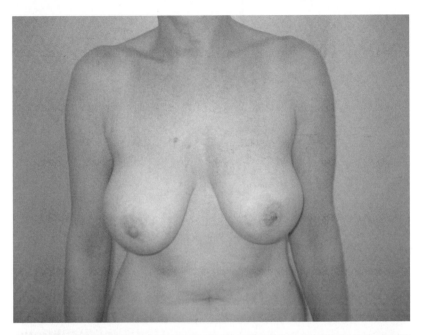

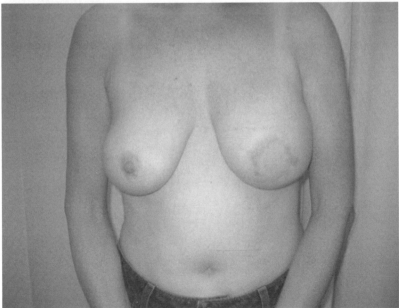

FIGURE 5.9 (top) Preoperative; (bottom) Postoperative left breast reconstruction with TDAP flap and implant, front view.

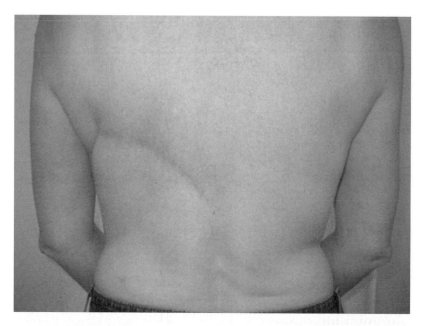

FIGURE 5.9(continued) Postoperative left breast reconstruction with TDAP flap and implant, back view.

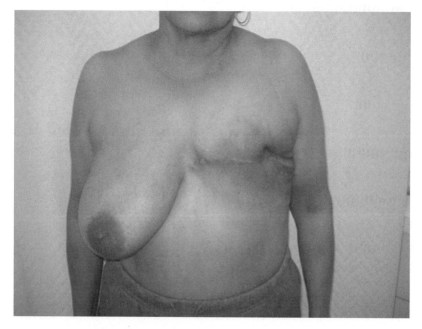

FIGURE 5.9(continued) Preoperative left breast reconstruction with latissimus dorsi flap and implant (Patient had post-mastectomy infection and radiation therapy in the past).

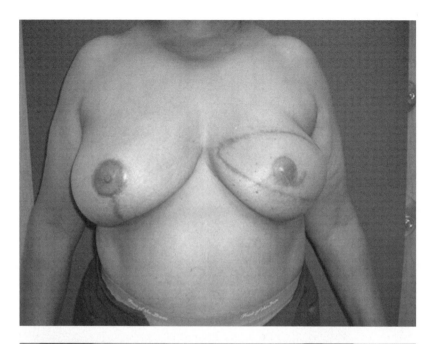

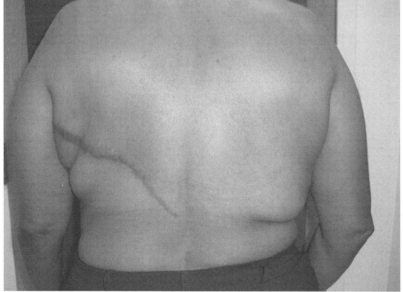

FIGURE 5.9(continued) Postoperative left breast reconstruction with latissimus dorsi flap and implant; (top) front view, (bottom) back view

Free TRAM Reconstruction

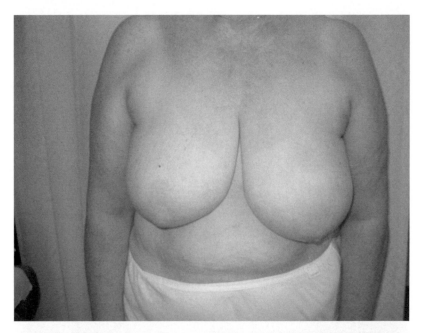

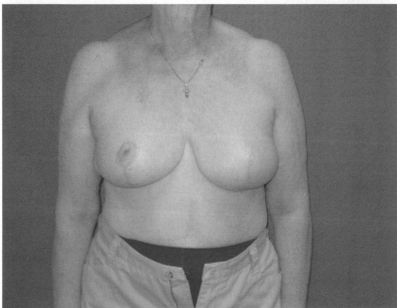

FIGURE 5.10 (top) Left free TRAM. (bottom) Right breast reduction for symmetry.

DIEP Reconstruction

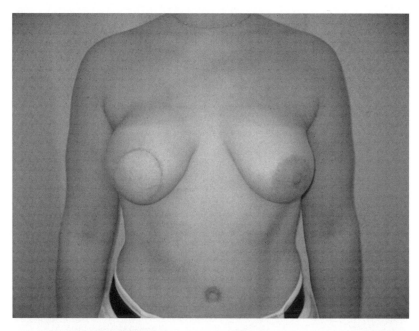

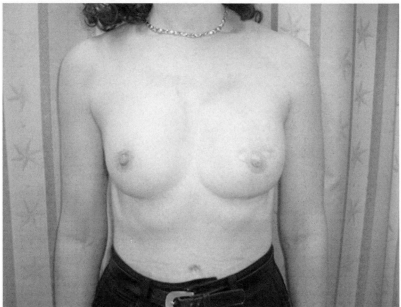

FIGURE 5.11 (top) Right DIEP flap. (bottom) Left DIEP flap.

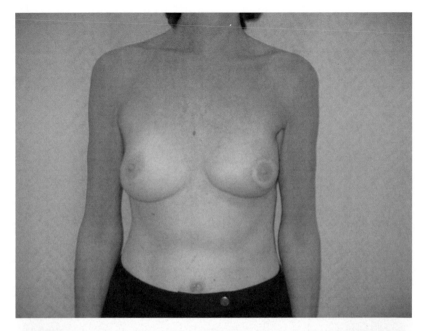

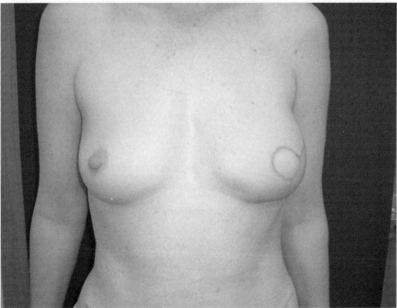

FIGURE 5.11(continued) (top) Left DIEP flap. (bottom) Left DIEP flap.

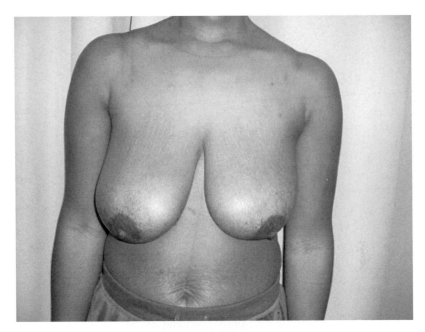

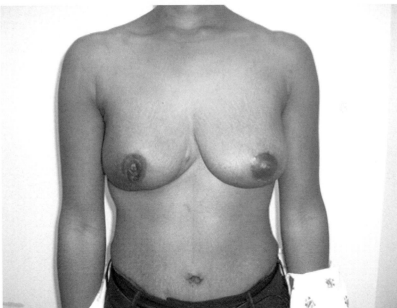

FIGURE 5.12 (top) Preoperative; (bottom) Right DIEP with left breast reduction.

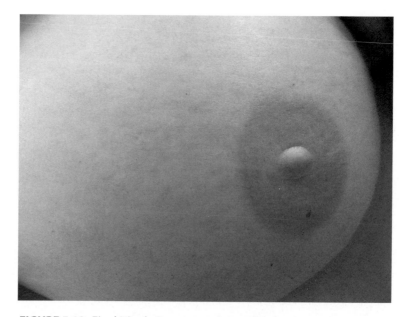

FIGURE 5.13 Final Nipple Reconstruction and Tattoo

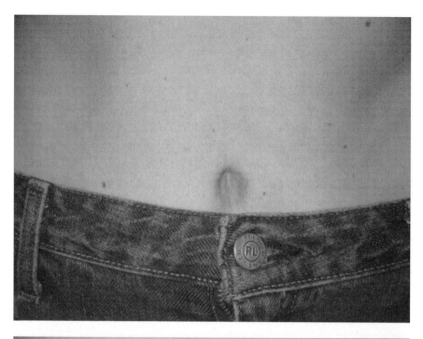

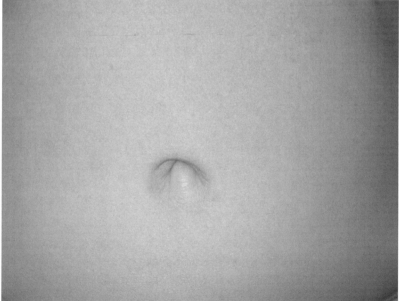

FIGURE 5.14 Close-up of umbilical reconstruction.

RISK FACTORS ASSOCIATED WITH POOR OUTCOMES

Smoking constitutes a constant threat to the patient's welfare—the risks for lung cancer, CAD, and peripheral vascular disease, among other conditions, are well known. A patient may be noncompliant with a physician's recommendation and/or smoking cessation program, and as a responsible adult she can make that informed refusal based on properly disseminated and properly received advice and data.[5]

However, when it comes to reconstruction of the breast—which is not an emergent or urgent condition—the patient has to understand that her chances of having a poor outcome are greater if she continues to smoke or to be exposed to nicotine in other forms. Whereas a patient may not stop smoking because of indifference to a silent, remote risk of hypertension and other pathological conditions, she is more likely to respond to an immediate cause-and-effect risk of a poor or failed outcome in breast reconstruction.

It is recommended that the patient be nicotine free for at least 6 weeks before reconstructive surgery—whether it is implant based or autologous tissue based. And by nicotine free, we mean the patient should have transitioned from smoking to patch or gum to nothing by the time of surgery. Whereas tobacco combustion products are noxious to the lungs, it is nicotine that is the critical agent in the vasoconstriction that leads to tissue ischemia.

Tissue ischemia, in turn, will cause fat necrosis with firm nodules in the reconstructed breast, abdominal wall delayed healing and necrosis, mastectomy flap necrosis, exposure and infection of the implants,[6] and, especially in conjunction with radiation, total flap necrosis. In addition to direct plastic surgery considerations, the higher rate of coughing in smokers can increase their risk for postoperative hernias in TRAM operations, prolonged recovery from anesthesia, and postoperative pneumonia.

The patient needs to understand that the precious resources of her body (e.g., abdominal skin and fat and back fat) will need to be conserved for use when the timing for reconstruction is optimal. To this end, her reconstructive surgery may even be cancelled if her urine nicotine test is positive (showing cumulative nicotine exposure for up to 4 weeks prior to surgery) or if an arterial blood gases (ABG) test shows elevated carboxyhemoglobin levels on the morning of surgery.

Some patients are surprised when during preoperative teaching they are informed that second-hand smoke exposure is just as deleterious as smoking itself.

Frequently patients with diabetes present for breast reconstruction. Because diabetes is a small-blood-vessel disease, it increases the rate of wound healing complications. For reconstructions in patients with diabetes, we undermine the abdomen less, transfer smaller amounts of tissue per perforator, or have to modify the technique to a muscle-sparing free TRAM to capture more blood vessels for the amount of tissue to be transferred. Blood sugar levels must be optimized before the time of surgery to mitigate the risk of infections for patients with diabetes.

CAD may influence the choice of vessels used for breast reconstruction. The recipient vessels where free flaps are transferred were traditionally the thoracodorsal artery and vein in the axilla. These vessels were often dissected and preserved during axillary dissections and easily accessible from the mastectomy defect.

With the change in oncologic surgery techniques, including skin-sparing mastectomy and lymph node sampling (sentinel lymph node), the vessels are neither accessible nor already dissected. In addition, because the risk of lymphedema increases with greater dissection in the axilla, and there is a concern that the oncologic surgeon may return to the axilla if the sentinel lymph node is positive, we want to avoid placing our delicate microanastomoses in the axilla. Furthermore, by leaving intact the thoracodorsals, which are the primary nutrient supply for the latissimus dorsi musculocutaneous flap and the TDAP flap, we save these vessels as future options for reconstruction if there is failure of the free flap.

Increasingly the choice of recipient vessels is the internal mammary (IM) artery and vein. These vessels are a good size-match for the deep inferior epigastric artery and vein, of a suitable caliber for microanastomoses (2–3 mm in diameter), and readily accessible in the center of the chest defect by resecting a 3-cm piece of the medial cartilaginous portion of rib 3 or 4. This allows the flap to be placed centrally to create a better-positioned breast mound, in contrast to the axillary anastomoses, which force the flap to be somewhat laterally situated. Occasionally we find perforators of the IM vessels arising from within the rib interspaces that, although smaller than the IM vessels themselves, are nonetheless usable for free-tissue transfer in our hands. The IM perforators are suitable for superficial inferior epigastric artery (SIEA) flap as well as DIEP flaps as much as 30% of the time. The preference for these vessels has to be communicated with the oncologic extirpative surgeon so that the vessels can be preserved during the mastectomy, as they arise at the lateral sternal border around ribs 2 to 4.[7]

The IM artery is the same vessel that cardiac surgeons use for coronary revascularization for patients with CAD. Arterial conduits, such as internal mammary artery–LIMA or radial artery grafts, have been shown to have a greater patency rate than saphenous vein grafts. Hence, cardiothoracic surgeons prefer a LIMA or occasionally a right internal mammary artery (RIMA) if it is available. Because our dissection utilizes the IM artery, the patient should be informed about the use of this vessel and its potential impact should she develop CAD. CAD may be more likely in the setting of radiation used to treat a left-sided breast cancer. Interestingly, breast cancer is slightly more common on the left than on the right. Our patients agree and request that their bodily resources be used to treat the disease that they currently have rather than a disease that they may or may not develop.[8]

Patients need to inform their cardiologist and cardiothoracic surgeons if in the future they need a coronary artery bypass graft (CABG) procedure. This information also needs to be disseminated to the cardiothoracic surgery literature. Occasionally, a left breast flap can be anastomosed to the right IM artery, and vice versa. Hence, simple visual inspection by the cardiothoracic surgeon will not suffice, and the surgeon should review the plastic surgery operative report.

THE SECOND STAGE AND CONTRALATERAL BREAST

Federal law requires that breast reconstruction be a covered benefit for women undergoing breast cancer management. This includes contralateral breast procedures to create symmetry and balance. Our goals in treating breast reconstruction are the "4 S's" of breast:

1. Size. The breast size should be appropriate to the woman's overall body habitus. This includes choosing an implant that will create an acceptable breast, but not so large that it threatens to attenuate the skin and cause local complications. For a flap, enough bulk has to be transported to create a mound of breast tissue.

2. Shape. To paraphrase Michaelangelo, "I saw an angel in the stone, and carved till I set it free." The bulk of autologous fat or implant has to be a teardrop–like shape, with good central projection, and roundness to the breast at the lower pole and a "ski slope" transition at the upper pole. This is achievable with either autologous tissue or with implants—especially shaped "contour" implants.

3. Sensuality. Ultimately the reconstruction should look attractive—that is, it should be sensual. Furthermore, it should eventually be sensate—capable of delivering both protective sensation and erogenous sensibility. Women have reported erogenous sensation from the reconstructed breast (personal communication, LS); this is feasible especially with skin-sparing mastectomies. Once the nerves reconnect, the signals they send to the brain are not the same as they were preoperatively, but how the brain is trained to interpret these signals is paramount. The largest sexual organ is between our ears—the brain. Sensations from our earlobes, fingers, neck, genitalia, thighs, and toes can be interpreted by our brains as sensual. Studies have shown that the more attractive the breast and donor site are, the more likely the breast will be perceived as sensual.

4. Symmetry. The two breasts are never symmetric to start with and they will not be symmetric in the end. Although they cannot be the same, we can reconstruct them to be similar. The goal is not simply to create two attractive breasts, but to create two similarly attractive breasts. This is achievable by offering women whose reconstructed breast cannot be made to match their native breast a symmetry operation on the normal breast. This may include a reduction, an implant augmentation, or a lift (mastopexy) of the normal breast; this can be a "silver-lining" in the dark cloud of breast cancer. Both breasts can be rejuvenated. The WHCRA (1998) includes coverage for surgery of the opposite breast to achieve symmetry. Surgery on the opposite breast does place scars on the external breast skin as well as internally. It is important to have a baseline mammogram of the normal breast to confirm that it is, indeed, normal. Internal scars on the normal breast can be confusing because calcifications may mimic or obscure a malignancy. This remains largely a theoretical concern, and clinical trials confirm that surgery on the opposite breast remains safe.

IMPLANT-BASED RECONSTRUCTION

The most common breast reconstruction technique combines expansion of the breast skin with use of a temporary tissue expander, followed by insertion of a permanent silicone or saline breast implant. This type of reconstruction requires two separate operations.

At the time of the patient's mastectomy, the surgeon inserts a tissue expander beneath the patient's skin and chest muscle. Through a tiny valve mechanism located inside the expander, the nurse practitioner periodically injects a salt-water solution to gradually fill the expander over several weeks or months. The patient may feel a sensation of stretching and pressure in the breast area during this procedure, but most women do not find that it is too uncomfortable. This process will begin usually 2 weeks after the mastectomy, once the drains are removed. This procedure stretches the skin and muscle to make room for a temporary implant, just like a woman's belly stretches during pregnancy. The process continues until the size is slightly larger than the other breast. After the skin over the breast area has stretched enough, the expander is removed in a second operation and a more permanent implant is inserted. Some expanders are designed to be left in place as the final implant. The nipple and the dark skin surrounding it, called the areola, are reconstructed in a subsequent procedure.

With impant-based reconstruction, you will be in the hospital overnight and will be able to go home the next day. Many reconstruction options require a surgical drain to remove excess fluids from surgical sites immediately following the operation. In most circumstances, these drains will remain in place for 1 to 2 weeks. If they are highly productive, they will stay in longer.

You are likely to feel tired and sore for a week or two after reconstruction. Most of your discomfort can be controlled by medication prescribed by your doctor.

FLAP RECONSTRUCTION

An alternative approach to implant reconstruction involves creation of a skin flap using tissue taken from other parts of the body, such as the abdomen, the back, or the buttocks. This type of operation will require you to stay in the hospital for 3 to 4 days. You will also have 3 to

4 surgical drains depending on whether one or two breasts are reconstructed. In most circumstances, these drains will remain in for 1 to 2 weeks. If they are highly productive, they will stay in longer.

The recovery time for flap reconstruction is 4 to 6 weeks.

TRAM Flap

In this type of flap surgery, the tissue remains attached to its original site, retaining its blood supply. The flap consists of the skin, fat, and muscle with its blood supply, and is tunneled beneath the skin to the chest, creating a pocket for an implant or, in some cases, creating the breast mound itself, without need for an implant.

DIEP/SIEA Flap, Latissimus Dorsi Flap, and SGAP Flap

Another flap technique uses tissue that is surgically removed from the abdomen, back, or buttock and then transplanted to the chest by reconnecting the blood vessels to new ones in that region. This procedure requires the skills of a plastic surgeon who is also experienced in microvascular surgery.

Regardless of whether the tissue is tunneled beneath the skin on a pedicle or transplanted to the chest as a microvascular flap, this type of surgery is more complex than skin expansion. Scars will be left at both the tissue donor site and at the reconstructed breast, and recovery will take longer than with an implant. Conversely, when the breast is reconstructed entirely with the patient's own tissue, the results are generally more natural and there are no concerns about a silicone implant. In some cases, the patient may have the added benefit of an improved abdominal contour.

Chemotherapy or radiation may be recommended by the surgical oncologist following the mastectomy. If the patient chooses to have these treatments, it will delay her secondary procedures by a few months.

FOLLOW-UP PROCEDURES

Most breast reconstruction involves a series of procedures that occur over time. Usually the initial reconstructive operation is the most complex. Follow-up surgery may be required to replace a tissue expander with an implant; to reconstruct the nipple and the areola; or to enlarge,

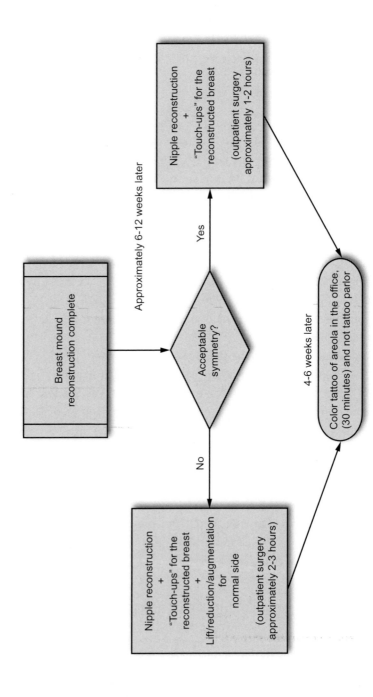

FIGURE 5.15 Outpatient "Touch-up" Surgeries

reduce, or lift the other natural breast to match the reconstructed breast. These secondary procedures are outpatient procedures and usually do not require the use of drains. The recovery time is based on the extent and complexity of the procedure, but usually ranges from a few days to a few weeks. (Figure 5.15)

Chances are that the reconstructed breast may feel firmer and look rounder or flatter than the natural breast. It may not have the same contour as the breast before mastectomy, and it will not exactly match the opposite breast. But these differences will be apparent only to the patient. For most mastectomy patients, breast reconstruction dramatically improves their appearance and quality of life following surgery.

ADVANTAGES AND DISADVANTAGES OF BREAST RECONSTRUCTION TECHNIQUES

DIEP/SIEA Flap Reconstruction

ADVANTAGES

▷ Because the reconstruction involves using the patient's own tissues, the risks of implant reconstruction are avoided.

▷ Most patients have less postoperative pain than after a TRAM flap and are, therefore, able to leave the hospital sooner and return to their normal activities more quickly than after a TRAM flap.

▷ Because abdominal muscle is not removed, patients have less risk of developing hernias at the site where the flap is removed than do patients who have had a TRAM flap.

▷ It is typically easier to match the contralateral natural breast with the patient's own tissue in flap reconstruction when compared with implant reconstruction.

▷ Patients essentially end up with a "tummy tuck" at the same time as the breast reconstruction.

DISADVANTAGES

▷ DIEP/SIEA flap reconstruction generally requires a longer and more difficult surgery at the first stage when compared with implants or TRAM flaps.

▷ Patients will have a scar across the lower abdomen where the flap is obtained.

Implant Reconstruction

ADVANTAGES

▷ The recovery from the initial expander placement surgery is usually quicker than for flap surgery.

▷ It may be easier to control the final size of the reconstructed breast with implant reconstruction.

▷ There are no scars on the patient's body other than those on the breasts.

DISADVANTAGES

▷ Because most patients require placement of an expander first followed by secondary replacement of the expander with an implant, at least two surgical stages are required as well as multiple visits to the plastic surgeon's office between these stages for tissue expansion.

▷ It is important to realize that for patients who are having a unilateral (one-sided) mastectomy, matching the other natural breast with an implant can be difficult. The shape and "feel" of an implant is not exactly like that of a natural breast.

▷ In the short term, implants can become infected or malpositioned and require surgery to correct these problems.

▷ In the longer term, implants can develop capsular contracture (tightening of the soft tissues around the implant), implant malposition, and implant rupture. All of these complications can require secondary procedures.

OTHER RECONSTRUCTION OPTIONS

The other breast reconstruction option is the latissimus flap, plus or minus an implant. This procedure leaves a scar across the patient's back, and would be used in conjunction with most likely a saline or silicone implant. The patient should understand that this procedure will lead to some loss of function with the latissimus dorsi, but this is not a dramatic functional loss for most people. With a pedicle flap, there is greater reliability in terms of flap healing but donor-site morbidity. In particular, seromas are fairly common in the latissimus dorsi donor site as well as a prominent scar.

With my patients, I also discuss the option of reconstruction using tissue from the patient's abdomen. She should understand that this could take the form of a pedicle TRAM flap, which harvests nearly the entire muscle and can leave her with weakness, bulging, or asymmetry. This option is less likely to have 100% failure, but there is a greater chance of fat necrosis associated with the pedicle flap especially in a patient with a heavyset body habitus.

Other flaps from the abdomen include a free TRAM flap, which involves microsurgery and transfer of a segment of the muscle as well as the overlying skin and fat. This is a good option and can decrease the risk of fat necrosis; however, there is a risk of weakness or bulge. The patient should understand that this flap can demonstrate an all-or-none phenomenon, with a complication resulting in loss of the entire flap as a possibility.

Another option for abdominal wall harvest is a free DIEP flap. This spares the muscle, but it is a lengthy and tedious dissection, which harvests skin and subcutaneous tissue but for the most part spares the muscle as well as the intercostal nerves. The patient should understand that this flap is associated with a higher risk of fat necrosis than is a free TRAM flap. However, the DIEP flap has a lower risk of abdominal wall weakness, bulge, or hernia. Moreover, this flap also demonstrates an all-or-none phenomenon. The flap complication rate is approximately 5% to 8%. If the patient were to have venous complications, she might require leech therapy and antibiotics as well as blood transfusions. If she were to have an arterial complication, she might require an urgent reoperation. Despite these measures, the flap might not be salvageable and total removal of the flap might be required. She might have to fall back on the other options, such as a latissimus flap plus or minus an implant, or tissue expander base reconstruction. It might not be possible to pursue these options at that same hospitalization.

In some anatomic scenarios, a DIEP flap may not be possible and the intraoperative alternatives would include conversion to a pedicled TRAM flap or implants.

Tissue expansion reconstruction is another possibility. This would involve placement of a saline or silicone tissue expander, which would require serial augmentation in the office over multiple visits spanning about 6 to 8 weeks. Once an adequate volume is reached, this implant would be removed and replaced with a permanent implant, either silicone or saline depending on the patient's preference. Implants have the risk of capsular contracture and rupture. The patient should understand that with implant reconstruction there is a higher rate of complications in the face of radiation should she require radiation postoperatively or if she has had radiation preoperatively.

～ Frequently Asked Questions

1. Will my breast and nipples have sensation?

In implant-based reconstruction, the nerves will reorient from the periphery and innervate the skin flaps from the edges. The ultimate innervation density will never be equivalent to the original, but protective sensation is obtained. However, no deeper nerves can migrate to the surface because of the presence of the artifical prosethesis—the implant. In autologous techniques, nerves can connect from the deeper surface to the transferred fat and skin. This is facilitated when, specifically, we connect a sensory branch from the abdominal fat to an intercostal nerve in the chest.

2. Are silicone implants safe?

Yes. In 2006, the U.S. Food and Drug Administration (FDA) approved silicone implants for use in cosmetic patients, and it had always allowed them for breast cancer reconstruction. No evidence of systemic disease caused by silicone implants has been found.[9] Because they are man-made objects and can rupture, the FDA recommends surveillance MRI scans every other year.

3. I have had prior surgery on my abdomen. Am I still a candidate for a flap?

Women who have had prior abdominal surgery, including cosmetic surgery, may not be candidates for reconstruction using abdominal tissue. For instance, an abdominoplasty (tummy tuck) precludes a TRAM, free TRAM, DIEP, or SIEA flap. Abdominal liposuction is not an absolute contraindication if the patient has regained the fatty deposits around the abdomen. If there is not sufficient fat in the subcutaneous tissues of the infraumbilical abdomen, then the patient is not a good candidate based on being thin, not based on prior liposuction.

Occasionally an appendectomy, hysterectomy, or cesarean section incision may have damaged the underlying blood vessels; however, this is usually not an issue. Prior open cholecystectomy scars can interefere with abdominal incision healing after a TRAM, free TRAM, DIEP, or SIEA flap, especially in patients who are obese [body mass index (BMI) greater than 30]. However, we do recommend a 3D CT perforator scan of the abdomen in patients who have had abdominal liposuction.

4. *Is breast reconstruction dangerous?*

No. Studies have demonstrated no increased rate of tumor recurrence, no delay in diagnosis, and no difference in overall survival in women who choose breast reconstruction versus those who choose no reconstruction. If the patient has many medical or psychological comorbidities, it may be prudent to wait for delayed reconstruction.

Prior or future planned radiation is a relative contraindication to implant-based reconstruction. Advanced age alone is not a contraindication.

We educate patients about these risks, which include, but are not limited to, infection, bleeding, pain, scarring, asymmetry, numbness, deformity, hypertrophic/keloid scarring, loss of nipple, poor healing, delayed healing, contour irregularity, abdominal wall bulge/weakness/hernia, interference with mammography and cancer surveillance, inability to breastfeed, financial risks, chronic pain, weakness, wound dehiscence, donor-site morbidity, need for additional surgery (planned or unplanned and emergent), and stiffness. We discuss the best-, average-, and worst-case scenarios related to the proposed surgery. We also discuss alternative methods of management, expected time and course of recovery, expected course of management of complications, and warning signs and symptoms of postoperative complications. We also talk about how radiation affects surgery, especially increasing the risks of complications. We further discuss diabetes, either diagnosed or undiagnosed, and how it may influence the outcome.

MANAGING COMPLICATIONS

Complications associated with implant-based reconstruction include

▷ Infection. Any prosthetic-based reconstruction is inherently at higher risk for infection, because the body cannot effectively clear bacterial attachment from the biofilm formed on artificial surfaces.[10] Infection is most likely in the perioperative period, but delayed infections can arise if the patient is bacteremic from another source such as an odontogenic infection or urinary tract infection. A trial of antibiotics (oral or intravenous, depending on the severity) is warranted, and if conservative management fails, explantation may be necessary. Typically a new implant cannot be placed at the same time and requires a "cooling off" period before another attempt at implant reconstruction can be considered, usually 2 to 3 months after explantation. There are some preliminary reports suggesting that antibiotic irrigation of the cavity with transfer of a muscle may allow immediate replacement with an implant.[11]

▷ Exposure/extrusion. In attenuated skin, especially in the setting of prior radiation, the mechanical pressure from the expander or implant can result in extrusion through the skin. When this happens, an area of surrounding tissue must be excised.

▷ Capsular contracture. Although the etiology of this in unclear and attributed to either hematoma during surgery, low-grade bacterial colonization, or an idiopathic process, capsular contracture may develop in the months to years after surgery.[12] A normal capsule develops around all implants, but a capsular contracture is defined as a scarring process that distorts the reconstruction and/or makes it painful. The rate of capsular contracture is reported as 8% to 20%. Fibrosis from radiation therapy is similar to capsular contracture and can similarly distort the breast. The Baker–Gordon classification for capsular contracture is as follows:

> Grade I: feels like normal breast tissue
>
> Grade II: somewhat firm but normal in appearance
>
> Grade III: firm and looks abnormal
>
> Grade IV: firm, painful, and deformed in appearance

▷ Rupture/deflation. Saline implants may rupture, and if this happens the implant deflates and the saline is harmlessly absorbed by the body. The outer shell then needs to be removed and replaced with a new implant. If a silicone implant ruptures, the rupture may go undetected because the silicone gel remains in the normal capsule that develops around the implant. The most sensitive study to evaluate rupture is magnetic resonance imaging (MRI). Even if the implant ruptures, surgery to remove the gel material and replace with a new implant is predictable and scientific studies have not demonstrated any systemic risk of disease related to silicone. In fact, in late 2006 the FDA approved silicone gel implants for use in cosmetic cases in addition to the existing allowance of using gel implants in reconstruction cases. The newer generation of silicone gels are "cohesive" or "memory gels" that are less likely to extrude the contents of the implants, even when ruptured.

Complications associated with flap reconstruction include

▷ Fat necrosis. After a flap is transferred, either as a pedicled or a free flap, there may be areas of fat that are underperfused. They will typically necrose and form firm nodules. Observation for a period of one year is warranted because much of this tissue softens during the postoperative interval. Firm nodules of fat necrosis feel quite different from tumor, but definitive diagnosis may require further imaging such as MRI or position emission tomography (PET) scan, or biopsy. Fat necrosis may also need to be excised if it is painful.

▷ Donor-site seroma.

▷ Total or partial flap loss.

5. *Does breast reconstruction affect breast cancer recurrence?*

Reconstruction has no known effect on the recurrence of disease in the breast, and it does not generally interfere with chemotherapy or radiation treatment, should cancer recur. Your surgeon may recommend continuation of periodic mammograms on both the reconstructed breast and the remaining normal breast. If your reconstruction involves an implant, be sure to go to a radiology center where technicians are experienced in the special techniques required to get a reliable x-ray of a breast reconstructed with an implant.

6. How will radiation affect my reconstruction?

The effects of radiation therapy on a reconstructed breast are unpredictable. Radiation affects every patient differently, but can cause hyperpigmentation due to burns, and changes in the texture and quality of the skin.[13] Some patients who desire to use their own tissue for reconstruction will have a tissue expander placed at the time of their mastectomy, undergo radiation treatment, and then at a later date have the expander removed and the breast recreated using their own tissues. This prevents the soft reconstructed breast from undergoing changes from radiation.[14]

Some studies have shown that patients who have radiation therapy are at an increased risk for problems with permanent implants.[15] These problems include capsular contracture, infection, and wound healing difficulties, causing loss of the implant. Discuss these options with your surgical oncology and plastic surgery team.

REFERENCES

1. Granzow JW, Levine JL, Chiu ES, Allen RJ. Breast reconstruction using perforator flaps. J Surg Oncol. 2006; 94:441–454.
2. Serletti JM. Breast reconstruction with the TRAM flap: Pedicled and free. J Surg Oncol. 2006;94:532–537.
3. Elliott LF, Hartrampf CR Jr. Breast reconstruction: Progress in the past decade. World J Surg 1990;14:763–775.
4. Spear SL, Mardini S, Ganz JC. Resource cost comparison of implant-based breast reconstruction versus TRAM flap breast reconstruction. Plast Reconstr Surg 2003;112:101–105.
5. Spear SL, Ducic I, Cuoco F, Hannan C. The effect of smoking on flap and donor-site complications in pedicled TRAM breast reconstruction. Plast Reconstr Surg 2005;116:1873–1880.
6. Cunningham M, Bunn F, Handscomb K. Prophylactic antibiotics to prevent surgical site infection after breast cancer surgery. Cochrane Database Syst Rev 2006;19:CD005360.

7. Rosson GD, Holton LH, Silverman RP, et al. Internal mammary perforators: A cadaver study. J Reconstr Microsurg 2005;21:239–242.

8. Nahabedian MY, Dooley W, Singh N, Manson PN. Contour abnormalities of the abdomen after breast reconstruction with abdominal flaps: The role of muscle preservation. Plast Reconstr Surg 2002;109:91–101.

9. Disa JJ, McCarthy CM. Breast reconstruction: A comparison of autogenous and prosthetic techniques. Adv Surg 2005;39:97–119

10. Spear SL, Carter ME, Schwarz K. Prophylactic mastectomy: Indications, options, and reconstructive alternatives. Plast Reconstr Surg 2005;115: 891–909.

11. Spear SL, Howard MA, Boehmler JH, et al. The infected or exposed breast implant: Management and treatment strategies. Plast Reconstr Surg 2004;113:1634–1644.

12. Wong CH, Samuel M, Tan BK, Song C. Capsular contracture in subglandular breast augmentation with textured versus smooth breast implants: A systematic review. Plast Reconstr Surg 2006;118:1224–1236.

13. Spear SL, Ducic I, Low M, Cuoco F. The effect of radiation on pedicled TRAM flap breast reconstruction: Outcomes and implications. Plast Reconstr Surg 2005;115:84–95.

14. Kronowitz SJ, Kuerer HM. Advances and surgical decision-making for breast reconstruction. Cancer 2006;107:893–907.

15. Behranwala KA, Dua RS, Ross GM, et al. The influence of radiotherapy on capsule formation and aesthetic outcome after immediate breast reconstruction using biodimensional anatomical expander implants. J Plast Reconstr Aesthet Surg 2006;59:1043–1051. Epub 2006 Jun 12.

Algorithm for Chemotherapy for Breast Cancer

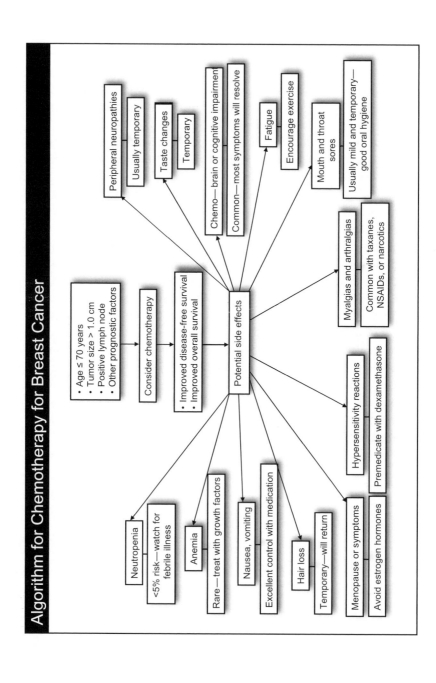

6

Chemotherapy for Breast Cancer

Carol Riley, CRNP
Deborah Armstrong, MD

What you need to know:

Chemotherapy may be administered to your patient prior to surgery—to shrink the tumor and provide a systemic treatment effect—or after surgery. Chemotherapy is used increasingly as the first defense against breast cancer (known as neoadjuvant chemotherapy), even for tumors that may be smaller, so as to measure tumor response and predict overall clinical outcome.

Women fear chemotherapy more than probably any other part of their breast cancer treatment.

Patients need to be in relatively good health prior to starting chemotherapy. Patients need to see you before starting their treatment to address routine health maintenance issues. The medical oncologist does not usually play this role.

Be sure your patient is up-to-date on the following health needs before starting chemotherapy: flu shots, dental work including cleanings, and no surgical procedures unless approved by her oncologist (even minor surgery).

Instruct your patient to continue to take her prescribed medications during chemotherapy. Advise her to not take supplements, vitamins, or herbal preparations without the oncologist's permission.

Many women are able to and choose to continue to work during chemotherapy.

Most side effects are manageable. (See the chart on page 108 for a summary). If you are prescribing something for your patient in response to her complaints about specific side effects, contact her medical oncologist to discuss this medication and make him or her aware of the problem.

What your patient needs to know:

Chemotherapy may be administered before or after surgery. The decision regarding the need for chemotherapy is based on histopathologic features of the tumor known from biopsy and from breast imaging studies, and from other possible staging information.

When chemotherapy is administered before surgery, the patient and her doctors can actually see how effective the drugs are in specifically destroying her cancer cells because the tumor in the breast will get smaller 40% of the time.

It is natural to be fearful of the side effects from chemotherapy. However, side effects are better controlled and prevented today than ever before.

Your patient needs a physical examination by her family doctor before starting chemotherapy so that her general health is assessed and preventive care is provided. This includes getting a flu shot (if it is flu season) as well as seeing her dentist for cleaning and any dental work that is needed.

The patient should not take vitamins, supplements, or herbal preparations without her oncologist approving them in advance, as little is known about drug interactions and these supplements may have a negative effect on the chemotherapy treatments.

The patient needs to inform her oncologist of any symptoms or side effects she is having so that they can be adequately treated as they occur. Self-medication without prior approval is to be discouraged.

Hair loss occurs with some of the more common treatment regimens. Getting fitted for a wig in advance is wise to consider. Hair loss occurs between days 14 and 17 after the first dose. The patient should request a prescription from her oncologist for a "cranial prosthesis" so that it can be submitted for reimbursement by her insurance company. Many insurers will cover this expense. (It is not covered if it is recorded on the prescription as a "wig.")

After hair loss, nausea and vomiting are the most common side effects women fear. Most women today do not experience this problem with the use of prophylactic antiemetics.

Exercise is a good way to combat fatigue.

Blood work will be done at specific intervals to monitor your patient's white blood cell and red blood cell counts. She needs to inform her doctor immediately if she develops a high fever. She should also avoid being around people who are sick with respiratory illnesses such as a cold or flu. Routine handwashing is a good practice to reduce risk of infection.

Cognitive impairment, known as "chemo brain," is being studied rigorously to understand its cause and learn how to reduce the incidence. It should not deter the patient from agreeing to chemotherapy, when recommended as part of her treatment.

INTRODUCTION

The goals of chemotherapy are to prevent or stop the growth of microscopic cancer cells to reduce the risk of recurrent or metastatic disease. The decision to treat with chemotherapy is individualized and is based on prognostic factors such as the tumor size and the number of lymph nodes involved. Chemotherapy has been shown to improve the long-term, relapse-free, and overall survival in women up to age 70 years regardless of nodal status.

The National Comprehensive Cancer Network (NCCN) guidelines recommend that women with a tumor size greater than 1 cm or those with node-positive disease be considered for chemotherapy.[1]

There are many proven chemotherapy options available (see Table 6.1). Chemotherapy may be given prior to the final surgery—known as preoperative, neoadjuvant, or primary chemotherapy—or after surgery has been completed. Any of these methods is appropriate and none at this point appears to have a survival advantage. Historically preoperative chemotherapy was used for patients with large tumors with the goal of downstaging the tumor size to allow for breast conservation. More recently, there has been more interest and research in primary chemotherapy with the goal of determining tumor response and predicting overall outcome.

Chemotherapy is one of the most feared aspects of treatment for breast cancer. Many women are concerned how treatment will affect

TABLE 6.1   ～   Common Chemotherapy Regimens

Chemotherapy	Administration schedule
(AC) Doxorubicin 60 mg/m² Cyclophosphamide 600 mg/m²	AC x4 →surgery →AC x4 AC x6–8 →surgery Surgery →AC x4
Paclitaxel 175 mg/m² or Docetaxel 100 mg/m²	AC x4 →surgery → taxane Taxane x4 →surgery →taxane (x4) Surgery→AC x4→taxane x4
(FAC) 5-Fluorouracil 600 mg/m² Doxorubicin 60 mg/m² Cyclophosphamide 600 mg	FAC x4 →surgery →FAC x4 FAC x6–8 →surgery surgery→FAC x6–8
(FEC) 5-Fluorouracil 600 mg/m² Epirubicin 50 mg/m² Cyclophosphamide 600 mg/m²	FEC x4→surgery →taxane x4 FEC x4–8 →surgery FEC x4→surgery →FEV x4

their relationships, their ability to care for their children, and their responsibilities at work. However, treatment today is much more tolerable than it was in the past, primarily because of the medications available to manage the side effects of treatment.

PREPARING FOR CHEMOTHERAPY

Feeling prepared when starting chemotherapy gives women a sense of control and will help reduce anxiety levels. The Internet alone can provide a wealth of information; unfortunately, much of this information is false, misleading, or confusing at best.

Women should be directed to their doctor or nurse for specific information regarding their treatment, the side effects of treatment, and the management of symptoms. Women should also limit their information gathering to reputable sources such as the American Cancer Society.

It is important for women to be in good health before beginning chemotherapy. Women should have a primary care doctor who will manage other health problems and screen for routine health maintenance before, during, and after chemotherapy. Women should not count on their oncologist to provide evaluation of or treatment for other health issues. Coexisting conditions such as high blood pressure and diabetes should be in good control before and during chemotherapy. For specific or particularly difficult health conditions, the oncologist may wish to consult the primary doctor.

Other general considerations are listed as follows:

▷ Vaccinations should be up-to-date, including the flu vaccine if the patient is undergoing chemotherapy during flu season. The pneumonia vaccination may be given if patients are considered to be at risk for this disease because of age or other health conditions.

▷ Dental work, including cleanings, should be done before chemotherapy and should be avoided during treatment. If a dental emergency should arise, consult with the oncologist before undergoing any procedure.

▷ No surgical procedures, no matter how small, should be done during chemotherapy without first talking to the oncologist.

▷ Patients should plan on taking any previously prescribed medications during chemotherapy, but should first check with the oncologist.

▷ Patients should not take any supplements, vitamins, or herbal preparations without first talking to the oncologist.

WORKING DURING CHEMOTHERAPY

Depending on the treatment plan and how each individual patient tolerates treatment, most women are able to work during chemotherapy. For some women it is important to maintain some normalcy and continue to be mentally active. Others choose to take time off to concentrate on their health. Many women are able to work a modified schedule. Women should check with their benefit plan and with their boss to determine what benefits and/or flexibility they may be allowed in their workday.

SIDE EFFECTS OF CHEMOTHERAPY

Side effects of chemotherapy are usually not life-threatening, vary in degree, and typically follow a predictable course. According to the Eastern Cooperative Oncology Group (ECOG) grading system, side effects are measured on a scale from 0 to 4, with 0 being normal and 4 being the most severe or life-threatening. Severe side effects can cause a delay in therapy, a dose modification of the drug(s), or cessation of therapy. Patients are monitored closely during chemotherapy and any unacceptable side effects may warrant any one of these changes.

Side effects of breast cancer treatment vary depending on the specific chemotherapy regimen. However, common side effects include hair loss, nausea, vomiting, taste changes, mouth sores, myalgias and arthalgias, hypersensitivity reaction, fatigue and peripheral neuropathy, neutropenia, anemia, and premature menopause.

Hair Loss

Most, but not all, regimens of chemotherapy cause hair loss. Most women will lose all of their scalp hair as well as eyebrows, eyelashes, and pubic hair. Hair loss usually occurs about 14 to 17 days after the first dose of chemotherapy. Many patients have mild scalp tenderness just before hair loss begins.

Most patients wear wigs, turbans, scarves, or hats. Fortunately, many insurance companies will pay for a wig with a written prescription from the doctor or nurse practitioner. The prescription should read "cranial prosthesis," as it is not covered by insurance if requested as a "wig."

Hair growth will return after chemotherapy is completed, but the texture or color may be slightly different.

Nausea and Vomiting

Although many patients fear nausea and vomiting the most, there are a number of antinausea medications available to manage and control these side effects. Some common drugs used include Emend, Anzemet, Zofran, Kytril, Compazine, Decadron, and Ativan. These drugs work very well. Severe nausea is not expected, but may occur in rare circumstances.

Taste Changes

Taste changes are common during chemotherapy and may include a metallic or unpleasant taste in the mouth. Some patients find that food tastes differently and many may have food cravings. This is generally more noticeable the first few days after chemotherapy, but can often take a few months to completely dissipate.

Mouth and Throat Sores

Many patients develop some mouth sores during chemotherapy. This side effect is more common during the second week after treatment, and is usually mild and dissipates in a few days. Rarely patients have severe ulcers that cause pain and interfere with eating and swallowing.

Treatment for these mouth sores varies and can include commercial mouthwash, prescription mouthwash, or local pain relievers. Although rare, some patients may require systemic pain medication. It is important that patients be instructed to keep their mouth clean by brushing, flossing, and rinsing after each meal. Commercial mouthwash with alcohol should be avoided, because it may cause further irritation.

Thrush is a common occurrence among patients receiving chemotherapy, and patients should be taught to watch for and report any symptoms to the doctor or nurse immediately.

Myalgias and Arthralgias

Some chemotherapeutic agents, particularly the taxanes, can cause joint and muscle pain for a few days after chemotherapy. This is common and can be treated with over-the-counter anti-inflammatories. In some cases the pain may be more severe and require treatment with narcotics. Pain usually subsides within a few days to a week, but in some cases may last longer.

Hypersensitivity Reactions

Taxanes, taxol, and taxotere can produce an allergic or hypersensitivity reaction. To prevent or lessen the reaction, patients are premedicated with dexamethasone 12 and 6 hours before the infusion. If a reaction should occur, the drug is discontinued and patients are treated for the reaction with additional medications. In rare cases epinephrine is necessary. Most patients are able to resume therapy when administered at a slower rate.

Fatigue

Fatigue is common during breast cancer treatment and one of the most debilitating side effects. The severity may vary, but most women do experience fatigue at some point during or after treatment. The exact cause of fatigue during chemotherapy is unknown but certainly anemia may affect a patient's level of fatigue, so this will be monitored by the treating oncologist.

There has been a wealth of research on fatigue that supports the use of moderate exercise or physical activity during chemotherapy. A brisk walk for 15 to 30 minutes, 5 days a week, has been shown to improve physical fitness and allows patients to perform activities of daily living.[2, 3]

It is important for health care providers to explain the benefits of exercise and to encourage patients to increase physical activity to improve their overall health and well-being.

Peripheral Neuropathies

Certain chemotherapy medications can cause peripheral neuropathies. In general, this side effect is temporary and returns to normal in most patients once the treatment is completed. In some patients this side effect can be permanent, so careful evaluation and monitoring is important. A dose modification or a modification in the treatment schedule may be necessary to avoid permanent problems. If peripheral nueropathy does become a problem, treatment with medications, such as Neurontin, may help reduce the associated discomfort.

Neutropenia

Neutropenia occurs in fewer than 5% of patients undergoing adjuvant therapy for breast cancer. It generally occurs 7 to 14 days after treatment, but the timing varies depending on the drugs administered. In most patients, this does not represent a problem unless a febrile illness occurs.

Blood is not usually drawn for blood cell counts in between treatments unless patients present with fever or some other symptom. Once a febrile illness occurs, careful evaluation to determine the source of the fever with a chest x-ray, blood and urine cultures, and careful physical examination is warranted. More frequently, no obvious cause is determined and patients are treated empirically.

Patients who are considered low risk—those without comorbid conditions and in otherwise good health—are most often treated at home with oral antibiotics. The current NCCN guidelines recommend treatment with oral ciprofloxacin and Augmentin.

For patients who are considered high risk—those with comorbid conditions, such as HIV or autoimmune disease; the elderly; or those who have a documented source of infection—admission to the hospital for treatment with intravenous antibiotics is necessary.

Subsequent treatment with chemotherapy may require a dose reduction, a change in treatment schedule, or the addition of growth factors such as Neupogen or Neulasta if not already a part of the treatment plan.

Patients should be instructed to immediately report any potential symptoms of infection including:

▷ Fever higher than 100.5 °F
▷ Chills or shaking
▷ New cough or trouble breathing
▷ Burning or pain when urinating
▷ Redness, swelling, soreness, or drainage from any body part
▷ Chills or shaking after flushing the catheter

Although most infections are not acquired from other individuals, careful personal care is important. Patients should be taught the following:

▷ Frequent handwashing, especially before meals and after using the bathroom. Remind visitors to wash their hands. Waterless hand gel can be used when soap and water are not available.
▷ Clean your mouth after each meal and at bedtime.
▷ Bathe or shower daily using a mild soap. Moisturize to prevent cracks in your skin. Use care when trimming nails.
▷ Clean your rectal area gently and thoroughly after bowel movements. Do not use enemas or suppositories.
▷ Urinate after intercourse to reduce bladder infections and clean your genital area thoroughly. Use a condom to prevent infection. Do not use tampons; they may lead to infection.
▷ Wash all fruits and vegetables. Do not eat undercooked foods.
▷ Avoid people with obvious infections. However, it is not necessary to avoid children or crowds.
▷ Take your temperature once a day or anytime you feel warm or chilled.
▷ Do not clean cat litter boxes, bird cages, or fish or reptile tanks.

Anemia

Anemia is a rare complication of adjuvant treatment for breast cancer, but is seen more commonly in patients being treated chronically for metastatic disease. Patients' blood cell counts are monitored with each treatment, and although a blood transfusion is rare, treatment with growth factors such as darbopoetin or erythropoetin is common and very helpful. Lack of iron, vitamin B_{12}, and folic acid may also cause anemia, so their levels may be checked during chemotherapy as well. Patients may feel tired, dizzy, weak, or short of breath, and these symptoms should be reported to the doctor.

Cognitive Impairment (Chemo Brain)

It is estimated that 18% to 82% of cancer patients who receive standard-dose chemotherapy will develop some cognitive impairment. This includes memory loss, inability to concentrate, inability to perform multiple tasks, and others. Although most of these symptoms improve in just a few months after treatment, cognitive impairment has been observed for 2 years or longer after treatment was completed.

The exact cause is likely multifactoral—that is, chemotherapy, hormonal therapy, stress, depression, and menopause. Although patients have been complaining of this side effect for years, little is known about its exact cause, prevalence, or treatment. It has been only recently that cognitive impairment has begun being investigated. There are multiple ongoing trials that will answer some of these questions. This lack of knowledge is frustrating for patients; however, it is somewhat reassuring that most symptoms will completely resolve shortly after treatment is completed.[4]

Menopause or Menopausal Symptoms

Chemotherapy in premenopausal women can often cause women to enter menopause either permanently or temporarily. These women can experience premature menopausal symptoms, which can be psychologically and physically difficult. Evidence suggests that treatment with estrogen may increase the risk of breast cancer recurrence, so management of these symptoms becomes a challenge.[5] Many women have severe and sometimes debilitating hot flashes. There is evidence that selective serotonin reuptake inhibitors (SSRIs) such as venlafaxine, paroxetine, or fluoxetine may decrease hot flashes by 45% to 60%.

Another study reports that gabopentin may decrease the frequency and intensity of hot flashes.[6]

There have been few studies of herbal treatments with breast cancer patients. Randomized trials with soy products failed to demonstrate a significant improvement in hot flash symptoms when compared to placebo. Similar results were reported from a study randomizing breast cancer patients to black cohosh or placebo. The safety of these products has not been demonstrated for use in the breast cancer population, as the phytoestrogens may stimulate breast cancer and antagonize the antitumor effects of tamoxifen.[7]

Vaginal dryness is another common menopausal symptom that is difficult to manage. In some cases, it can be successfully treated with over-the-counter vaginal lubricants. In other patients, however, this does not relieve the symptoms and the use of local or topical estrogen therapy is very effective. However, some estrogen is systemically absorbed with this route, and there are no data to assess the safety of topical estrogen use in patients with breast cancer. Although the exact risk is not known, some women are willing to take on this risk to improve their quality of life.

Menopause combined with treatment with aromatase inhibitors can cause calcium loss from bones. The management of osteoporosis in women with breast cancer does not differ from that of women without breast cancer. Adequate dietary intake of calcium (1200 mg/day) and vitamin D (400–800 IU), regular exercise, and avoidance of smoking are recommended. Monitoring with a bone density scan and treatment with bisphosphonates should be instituted as necessary.

⁀ Frequently Asked Questions

1. *Can patients travel while undergoing chemotherapy? And if so, what precautions should be taken?*
   a. In most cases, yes, as long as patients are traveling to an area where good medical care can be received urgently if necessary. However, it is recommended that patients do not travel during their first cycle of chemotherapy, because at that point the side effects and tolerance of therapy are unknown.
   b. It is not necessary to wear a face mask during air travel.
   c. Frequent handwashing is essential.

    d. Wear loose-fitting, nonconstrictive clothing.

    e. Get up every 30 to 60 minutes and walk up and down the aisle of the plane.

    f. Drink plenty of fluid to avoid dehydration.

    g. The National Lymphedema Network (NLN) recommends that:

       1. Individuals with a **confirmed diagnosis** of lymphedema should use some form of compression therapy (i.e., compression garment or compression bandages) while traveling by air.

       2. Individuals **at risk** for developing lymphedema should understand the risk factors associated with air travel and should make a decision to use compression therapy based on their individual risk factors.[8]

2. *If a patient calls with a fever during chemotherapy, how should she be advised?*

    a. If they call during working hours, patients should be advised to notify their treating oncologist. In most circumstances, patients will be seen immediately for evaluation and treatment.

    b. If patients live more than 45 minutes away from the treating oncologist, they will be advised to see their primary medical doctor immediately during working hours or to go to the emergency room if after hours.

    c. Evaluation of a febrile patient (>100.5 °F) during chemotherapy includes the following:

       1. Blood work—complete blood count, comprehensive metabolic panel, blood cultures

       2. Urine cultures/culture of any other obvious source—that is, wound, central catheter site

       3. Chest x-ray or other imaging study as indicated

    d. Treatment depends on the laboratory values and clinical evaluation (see the section on neutropenia).

3. *My patient has completed her treatment with chemotherapy. What type of evaluation or scanning is involved?*

The National Comprehensive Cancer Network (NCCN) recommends the following guidelines:

a. Interval history and physical examination every 4 to 6 months for 5 years, then every 12 months.

b. Mammogram every 12 months (and 6 to 12 months post-radiation therapy if breast conserved).

c. No specific blood work or radiological evaluation needed unless otherwise recommended—that is, routine health maintenance.

d. Women on tamoxifen: annual gynecologic assessment every 12 months if the uterus is present.

e. Women on an aromatase inhibitor or who experience ovarian failure secondary to treatment: monitoring of bone health.

REFERENCES

1. National Comprehensive Cancer Network. Practice guidelines for breast cancer. Version 1, 2007; revised 11/09/06.

2. Mock V. Exercise manages fatigue during breast cancer treatment: A randomized controlled trial. Psycho-Oncology 2005;14:464–477.

3. Stricker CT. Evidenced-based practice for fatigue management in adults with cancer: Exercise as an intervention. ONF 2004;31(5):963–976.

4. Meyers CA, Abbruzzese JL. Cognitive functioning in cancer patients: Effect of previous treatment. Neurology 1992;42:434–436.

5. Rossouw JE, Anderson GL, Prentice RL, et al. Risks and benefits of estrogen plus progestin in healthy postmenopausal women: Principal results From the Women's Health Initiative randomized controlled trial. JAMA 2002;288:321–333.

6. Pandya KJ, Thummala AR, Griggs JJ, et al. Pilot study using gabapentin for tamoxifen-induced hot flashes in women with breast cancer. Breast Cancer Res Treat 2004;83:87–89.

7. Van Patten CL, Olivotto IO, Chambers GK, et al. Effect of soy phytoestrogens on hot flashes in postmenopausal women with breast cancer: A randomized controlled clinical trial. J Clin Oncol 2002;20:1449–1455.

8. National Lymphedema Network. Position statement of the National Lymphedema Network. 5/19/2004; review date: 5/19/2007.

Algorithm for Pharmacogenetics

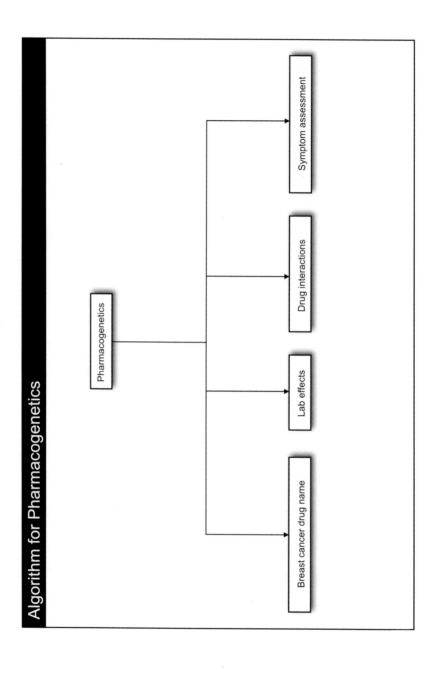

chapter

7

Pharmacogenetics and Breast Cancer Treatment

Lillie D. Shockney, RN, BS, MAS

What you need to know:

Women do not always realize that other medications or herbs/supplements they are taking may interfere with the drugs and therapies being given to them as part of their breast cancer treatment. Ask the patient about every drug, supplement, and even vitamin, she is taking; this is important baseline information to have for her medical record.

Patients will commonly ask their gynecologist or primary care provider (PCP) for "symptom relief" from drug side effects they are experiencing that are associated with hormonal therapy for breast cancer prevention or gastrointestinal side effects associated with chemotherapy or other drugs prescribed during their breast cancer treatment. Caution needs to be exercised before prescribing medications or even herbal options for these patients, as there may be contraindications to doing so.

What your patient needs to know:

Taking medications or herbal supplements without informing her doctors is unwise. Self-prescribing for symptom relief is also to be discouraged.

The patient should inform her doctor if she is having unpleasant side effects from a specific treatment so that he or she can appropriately prescribe something to help alleviate those side effects or direct the patient in another manner (such as exercising to counteract fatigue from radiation) to obtain symptom relief.

Some medications stay in the body for a long time. The patient needs to factor this in when considering adding other medications or supplements to her daily care program after she has completed a specific treatment regimen for her breast cancer.

INTRODUCTION

The purpose of this chapter is to provide information related to breast cancer drugs that a patient is currently taking and that may result in side effects, complications, or reduction in effectiveness if given with other prescription medications or supplements. Before beginning, however, some background information on the science of pharmacogenetics is provided here.

Pharmacogenetics is the study of how the actions of and reactions to drugs vary with the patient's genes, and specifically how people respond to drug therapies. Although this science is still considered fairly new, there have already been many useful discoveries. It has long been known that genes influence the risk of developing certain diseases, and that genes determine traits such as hair and eye color. Genes can also alter the risk for developing different diseases. In more recent years, research has discovered that genes can determine other aspects of the individual, down to the level of the enzymes produced in the liver. Because these enzymes determine how quickly a drug is excreted from the body, they can make major differences in the way people respond to drugs. Some of the most basic work concerns the way race and gender influence drug reactions—and race and gender are genetically determined. More specific research has identified individual genes that may influence drug response and drug interactions. Specific genes have been identified that may determine how patients will respond to specific drugs.

CAUSES AND SYMPTOMS

Genes alter responses to drugs because genes influence many parts of the body itself. For example, in the case of gender-related responses to antidepressant agents, women tend to show greater responses to serotonin-specific antidepressants because women naturally have lower levels of serotonin than men do. This makes women more likely to develop a type of depression marked by low serotonin levels, but it also means that women will respond better to replacement of serotonin.

Another trait that is influenced by genes is the production of a liver enzyme, CYP2D6. This enzyme metabolizes some drugs by converting them to a form that can be removed from the body. Genes determine the level of this enzyme in the liver. People with low levels of CYP2D6 will metabolize drugs slowly. Slow metabolism means the drugs will act for a longer period of time. Slow metabolizers respond to smaller doses of medications that are eliminated by this enzyme, whereas fast metabolizers—that is, people who have a lot of the enzyme—will need larger drug doses to get the same effects. At the same time, low levels of CYP2D6 mean that people taking the drugs that are metabolized by this enzyme will have higher drug levels and are more likely to experience undesired side effects.

Yet another mechanism of drug activity is the presence or absence of specific drug receptor sites. Drugs act by binding to specific chemicals, called receptor sites, within body cells. Genes may help determine how many of these cells there are. Other genetic studies indicate that genes may affect how people respond to foods as well as to drugs. An Australian study of osteoporosis, for example, reported that separate genes may affect a person's response to vitamin D, calcium, and estrogens.

IMPLICATIONS

Although studies in the field of pharmacogenetics promise to provide great benefits in drug effectiveness and safety, at the present time most drug treatment involves trial and error. That is, the physician prescribes a medication, and the patient takes the drug in good faith assuming that it will help whatever problem the drug is designed to medically address. The drug may work, or it may not. It may cause adverse effects, or it may be safe. If the drug does not work, the dose is increased. If the drug causes harmful or undesired side effects, a new drug might be tried until, finally, the right drug is found. In some cases, this process may take weeks or even months. In the case of cancer therapies, there may not be another drug to which to switch the patient, thereby creating the challenge of how to manage the side effects so the patient can reap the benefits of cancer therapy.

Table 7.1 on page 128 provides a list of the drug therapies most commonly given to breast cancer patients and women at high risk for breast cancer. Table 7.1 supplies the name of each drug, the class of the drug, the laboratory tests that are used to monitor the patient while taking that specific medication, and any medications or herbals/supplements that are contraindicated while the patient is taking the therapy.

〜 Frequently Asked Questions

1. *If a patient is taking hormone replacement therapy and is newly diagnosed with breast cancer, what instructions should she be given about coming off this drug?*

   What usually works best is having the patient wean off the medication. The "cold turkey" approach can be emotionally distressing, especially when added to a new diagnosis of breast cancer. The patient needs to begin by taking the medication every other day, then every third day, then twice a week, and so on, until the drug is discontinued. Remember that her cancer did not form overnight, so the medication so be stopped gradually, too. It is necessary to stop hormone replacement therapy in case of breast cancer, but this weaning should be accomplished over a 2- to 3-week period.

2. *Who is responsible for monitoring my patient's blood work while she is taking cancer medications that may affect her blood levels?*

   The doctor who prescribed the medications should be in charge of monitoring blood work the majority of the time; this provider is generally the patient's oncologist. However, if the patient is seeing you for a checkup or new onset of symptoms of some kind, it is appropriate to check her blood levels and contact her oncologist to make him or her aware of the results, whether they are abnormal or not.

3. **If the chart provided says there are no known drug interactions, is it safe to assume that whatever I might prescribe for the patient will not negatively affect her treatment?**

   Although that would be the hope, research is ongoing in this area; therefore, so it is prudent to stay abreast of updated reports that relate to the study of these drugs so that you will be aware of any new information that might affect your prescribing practices.

FURTHER READING

Kalow W (Ed.). *Pharmacogenetics of drug metabolism.* New York: Pergamon Press, 1992.

Novartis Foundation. *From genome to therapy: Integrating new technologies with drug development.* New York: John Wiley, 2000.

Wilkes GM. *Pocket guide to breast cancer drugs.* Sudbury, MA: Jones and Bartlett 2005.

ACKNOWLEDGEMENTS

The author would like to thank Dr. Vered Stearns, at Johns Hopkins, and Dr. James Rae at the University of Michigan, for their input to this chapter.

TABLE 7.1 ≈ Breast Cancer Drugs and Their Interactions

Drug Name	Class	Lab Effects/Interference	Drug Interactions
Anastrozole (Arimidex)	Nonsteroidal aromatase inhibitor	Elevated GGT	Currently unknown
Capecitabine (Xeloda)	Fluoropyrimidine carbamate	Increased bilirubin and alkaline phosphatase	Warfarin: increased INR, monitor and adjust dose prn Phenytoin: monitor phenytoin serum level closely and adjust dose prn Leucovorin: synergy and increased toxicity; monitor closely
Carboplatin (Paraplatin)	Alkylating agent	Increased LFT and RFT Monitor urine creatinine clearance	Cisplatin: combination may cause increased renal toxicity Myelosuppressive drugs: combination may cause increased bone marrow depression Taxol: carboplatin administered following taxol maximizes efficacy Avoid aluminum needles in drug handling
Cyclophosphamide (Cytoxan)	Alkylating agent	Increased potassium, uric acid secondary to tumor lysis Monitor electrolytes for symptoms of SIADH	Chloramphenicol: half-life may be increased Thiazide diuretics: combination can cause increased duration of leukopenia

Drug Name	Class	Lab Effects/Interference	Drug Interactions
		Decreased CBC and platelets	Anticoagulants: effects may be increased Digoxin: serum concentrations may be decreased and dose adjustments may be required Doxorubicin: cardiomyopathy may be potentiated Succinylcholine: may prolong neuromuscular blockage Barbiturates and other CYP450 inducers: increase cyclophosphamide activation and toxicity
Docetaxel (Taxotere)	Taxoid, mitotic spindle poison	Decreased CBC	Potential radiosensitization Inhibitors of CYP3A4: can decrease drug elimination and increase toxicity; caution should be observed
Doxorubicin hydrochloride (Adriamycin)	Anthracycline	Decreased CBC Increased LFT Increased uric acid secondary to tumor lysis	Barbiturates and other CYP450 inducers: may increase drug clearance Cyclophosphamide: combination may increase risk of hemorrhage and cardiotoxicity Mitomycin: combination may increase risk of cardiotoxicity

(continued)

TABLE 7.1 ≈ Breast Cancer Drugs and Their Interactions (*continued*)

Drug Name	Class	Lab Effects/Interference	Drug Interactions
Doxorubicin hydrochloride, lyposomal (Doxil)	Anthracycline	Decreased CBC	Digoxin: combination decreases digoxin serum concentrations Mercaptopurine: combination may increase risk of hepatotoxicity Heparin: incompatible due to precipitate formation No formal drug interactions reported; however, recommend same cautions as those for for Adriamycin
Epirubicin (Ellence, Farmorubicine, Farmorubicina, Pharmorubicin)	Anthracycline	Decreased WBC counts and neutrophil counts	Cytotoxic drugs: additive toxicity (hematologic and gastrointestinal) Cardioactive drugs: combination with calcium-channel blockers may increase risk of CHF; close cardiac function monitoring required Potential radiosensitization: given after radiation therapy; radiation recall inflammatory reaction may occur at site of prior radiation Cimetidine: combination increases drug AUC by 50%. *Do not use concurrently;* hold cimetidine during treatment.

Drug Name	Class	Lab Effects/Interference	Drug Interactions
Exemestane (Aromasin)	Steroidal aromatase inhibitor	Lymphopenia (20% incidence) Elevated LFT (AST, ALT, alkaline phosphatase, GGT) rarely	CYP450 inducers: may increase drug clearance
5-Fluorouracil (fluorouracil, Adrucil, 5-FU, Efudex)	Pyrimidine antimetabolite	Decreased CBC	Cimetidine: may increase pharmacologic effects of fluorouracil
Fulvestrant (Faslodex)	Estrogen-receptor downregulator	None	Currently unknown
Gemcitabine (Gemzar, difluorodeoxy-citidine)	Antimetabolite	Decreased CBC Increased LFT and RFT	Potential radiosensitization
Goserelin acetate (Zoladex)	Synthetic analog of luteinizing hormone-releasing hormone	Hypercalcemia in patients with bone metastasis	Currently unknown
Lapatinib (Tykerb)	Tyrosine kinase inhibitor	Monitor left ventricular function	CYP450 inhibitors and inducers: may alter metabolism

(continued)

TABLE 7.1 ～ Breast Cancer Drugs and Their Interactions (*continued*)

Drug Name	Class	Lab Effects/Interference	Drug Interactions
Letrozole (Femara)	Nonsteroidal aromatase inhibitor	Liver transaminases may be transiently elevated	Currently unknown
Leucovorin calcium (folinic acid, citrovorum factor)	Derivative of folic acid	None	5-Fluorouracil: potentiation Folic acid: can antagonize drug effect; high doses may decrease effects of phenobarbital, phenytoin, and primidone
Leuprolide acetate (Lupron, Viadur)	Antihormone	Decreased PSA, testosterone, WBC, and total serum protein; increased calcium; Injection: increased BUN and creatinine Depot injection: increased LDH, alkaline phosphatase, AST, uric acid, cholesterol, LDL, triglycerides, glucose, WBC count, phosphate; decreased potassium and platelets	
Megestrol acetate (Megace)	Synthetic progestin	Rarely, may increase glucose, LDH level	Currently unknown

Drug Name	Class	Lab Effects/Interference	Drug Interactions
Methotrexate (Amethopterin, Mexate, Folex, Trexall)	Antimetabolite, folic acid antagonist	Decreased CBC Increased LFT and RFT	Protein-bound drugs (aspirin, sulfonamides, sulfonylureas, phenytoin, tetracycline, chloramphenicol) may increase toxicity NSAIDs (including indomethacin and ketoprofen): may increase methotrexate serum concentration. *Do not administer concurrently with high doses of methotrexate; caution should be observed at moderate or low doses.* Cotrimoxazole and pyrimethamine: increase methotrexate serum levels; *do not use concurrently*
Mitoxantrone (Novantrone)	DNA intercalator	Decreased CBC Decreased electrolytes Increased LFT and uric acid	Myelosuppressive agents: combination can cause increased hematologic toxicity
Paclitaxel (Taxol)	Taxoid, mitotic inhibitor	Decreased CBC Increased LFT	Cisplatin: taxol should be given prior cisplatin to avoid decreased clearance and increased myelosuppression Ketoconazole and CYP3A4 inhibitors: may inhibit paclitaxel clearance; use together with caution

(continued)

TABLE 7.1 ～ Breast Cancer Drugs and Their Interactions *(continued)*

Drug Name	Class	Lab Effects/Interference	Drug Interactions
			Carboplatin: may increase cytotoxicity when administered after doxorubicin and liposomal formation: may increase incidence of neutropenia and stomatitis when administered after paclitaxel; combination may increase cardiotoxicity Beta blockers, calcium-channel blockers, and digoxin: additive bradycardia may occur; assess/monitor patient closely
Pamidronate disodium (Aredia)	Bisphosphonate	Decreased calcium, potassium, magnesium, and phosphorus levels	Caution indicated with nephrotoxins
Tamoxifen citrate (Nolvadex, Soltamox)	Antiestrogen	Decreased CBC Increased LFT and calcium levels Interference in lab tests as TFT and hyperlipidemia	Anticoagulants: increase PT; monitor PT closely and reduce anticoagulant dose CYP450 inhibitors and inducers: alter tamoxifen metabolism
Toremifene citrate (Fareston)	Synthetic tamoxifen analog	Decreased WBC and platelets	Testosterone and cyclosporine: may inhibit metabolism CYP450 inhibitors and inducers alter tamoxifen metabolism

Drug Name	Class	Lab Effects/Interference	Drug Interactions
			Thiazide diuretics: combination may increase risk of hypercalcemia
			Anticoagulants: increased PT; monitor PT closely and reduce anticoagulant dose
Trastuzumub (Herceptin)	HER2/neu antibody	Monitor left ventricular function	Paclitaxel: may inhibit elimination
Vinorelbine tartrate (Navelbine)	Semisynthetic vinca alkaloid	Decreased CBC (especially WBC count) Increased LFT	Cisplatin: combination may increase granulocytopenia
			Mitomycin: combination may increase acute pulmonary reactions
			CYP450 inhibitors: may alter metabolism; caution recommended when given concurrently
Zoledronic acid (Zometa)	Bisphosphonate	Hypocalcemia, hypophosphatemia, and hypomagnesemia Increased BUN and serum creatinine	Aminoglycoside antibiotics and loop diuretics: may potentiate hypocalcemia; caution recommended

ALT: alanine aminotransferase; AST: aspartate aminotransferase; AUC: area under the curve; BUN: blood urea nitrogen; CBC: complete blood count; CHF: congestive heart failure; DNA: deoxyribonucleic acid; GGT: gamma glutamyl transferase; INR: International Normalized Ratio; LDH: lactic dehydrogenase hormone; LDL: low-density lipoprotein; LFT: liver function tests; NSAIDs: nonsteroidal anti-inflammatory drugs; prn: *pro re nata* ("as needed"); PSA: prostate-specific antigen; PT: prothrombin time; RFT: respiratory function tests; SIADH: syndrome of inappropriate antidiuretic hormone; TFT: thyroid function tests; WBC: white blood cell

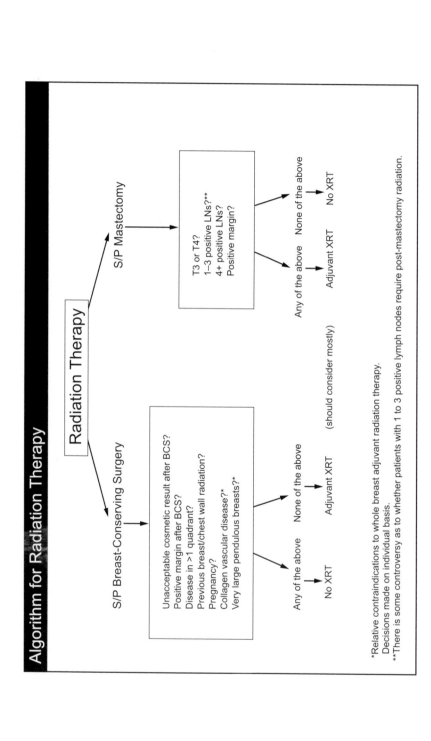

Algorithm for Radiation Therapy

Radiation Therapy

S/P Breast-Conserving Surgery

S/P Mastectomy

Unacceptable cosmetic result after BCS?
Positive margin after BCS?
Disease in >1 quadrant?
Previous breast/chest wall radiation?
Pregnancy?
Collagen vascular disease?*
Very large pendulous breasts?*

Any of the above — No XRT

None of the above — Adjuvant XRT   (should consider mostly)

T3 or T4?
1–3 positive LNs?**
4+ positive LNs?
Positive margin?

Any of the above — Adjuvant XRT

None of the above — No XRT

*Relative contraindications to whole breast adjuvant radiation therapy.
Decisions made on individual basis.
**There is some controversy as to whether patients with 1 to 3 positive lymph nodes require post-mastectomy radiation.

chapter

8

Radiation Therapy for Breast Cancer

Richard C. Zellars, MD

What you need to know:

Breast-conserving surgery followed by whole-breast radiation is equivalent to mastectomy for the majority of women with early-stage breast cancer.

The local failure rate at 5 years after breast-conserving surgery followed by radiation is less than 10%; the corresponding rate for breast-conserving surgery without subsequent radiation is 30% to 40%. Approximately 75% of local failures occur within the first 5 years after breast-conserving therapy.

Absolute contraindications to breast-conserving therapy include the following conditions:

▷ Positive margins after conservative surgery

▷ A cosmetically unacceptable result after conservative surgery

▷ Previous breast/chest wall radiation therapy

▷ Pregnancy

▷ Disease in more than one quadrant of the breast

Relative contraindications include collagen vascular disease and extremely large, pendulous breasts.

Tattoos and nonpermanent marks are placed on the skin to assist with daily positioning for radiation therapy. Patients should be discouraged from removing these tattoos, as they serve as important marks if the patient ever needs radiation to the contralateral breast.

Postmastectomy radiation has been shown in randomized prospective trials to improve survival for women with one to three positive nodes (controversial) and four or more positive nodes (widely accepted).

Radiation side effects may include the following:

▷ Early effects: fatigue, skin irritation, and breast edema.
▷ Late effects: breast shrinkage, breast edema, fibrosis, hypopigmentation or hyperpigmentation, and tenderness. Radiation pneumonitis is characterized by dry, nagging cough.

What your patient needs to know:

Radiation after lumpectomy maximizes local control for the majority of women with breast cancer.

A typical course of adjuvant whole-breast radiation therapy lasts 5 to 7 weeks. In the first 5 weeks or so, the entire breast is treated. Typically, during the remaining 2 weeks, an extra dose of radiation is delivered to the lumpectomy site.

Partial-breast irradiation, which would allow for a shorter course of radiation, is currently under both national and international investigation. Partial-breast irradiation may be delivered via external beam radiation therapy or by placing a radioactive source through the breast or in the lumpectomy cavity. These treatments have not been proven to be equivalent to standard whole-breast radiation.

Tattoos are permanent and are used for ensuring that the correct area is irradiated. These tattoos should not be removed, as they are important in the event that radiation to the other breast is ever needed.

Radiation, like surgery, is a local therapy.

Skin irritation, appearing like a sunburn, and fatigue are not uncommon in women who receive radiation therapy. Radiation has cumulative effects, so these side effects may worsen during the course of therapy.

The patient should review with the radiation oncologist the risks of lung and heart damage from the proposed course of radiation.

Nausea and vomiting are extremely uncommon with breast radiation therapy. Likewise, the patient will not lose the hair on her head due to breast irradiation.

~ ~ ~

INTRODUCTION

Radiation oncology is integral to the management of breast cancer. The majority of breast cancer patients will have some meaningful interaction with a radiation oncologist at some point during their care. The purpose of this chapter is to give the non-oncology health care provider a primer on radiation therapy in breast cancer.

Radiation works by disrupting the DNA of both cancer cells and normal cells. Normal cells with intact DNA repair mechanisms are able to correct this damage. Cancer cells, which often lack intact DNA repair mechanisms, are unable to correct the DNA damage and as a result are preferentially killed. To maximize the differential killing of these cells while minimizing damage to normal cells, it is necessary to deliver the radiation over several days to weeks; this process is called fractionation. By fractionating the treatment, the noncancerous cells have time to repair the DNA damage before the next round of radiation treatment.

INVASIVE BREAST CANCER

Breast-Conserving Therapy

The most common use of radiation with respect to breast cancer is in relation to breast-conserving therapy (BCT). To date, there have been seven randomized prospective trials comparing mastectomy to limited breast surgery (lumpectomy) with or without adjuvant whole-breast radiation.[1,2] These trials not only showed that there was similar survival between mastectomy and lumpectomy patients, but also demonstrated that whole-breast irradiation after lumpectomy significantly reduces the incidence of local failures when compared to patients treated with lumpectomy alone. As a result, the National Cancer Institute (NCI) put forth this consensus statement:

> Breast conservation treatment is an appropriate method of primary therapy for the *majority* of women with stage I–II breast cancer and is preferable because it provides survival rates equivalent to those of total mastectomy and axillary dissection while preserving the breast.

If the majority of women with early-stage breast cancer are eligible for BCT, who are the minority of women for whom BCT is not an option? In other words, what are the contraindications to BCT? These contraindications can be classified into three general categories: unacceptable cosmetic result, complication rate, and recurrence rate. Next, we discuss each of these categories briefly.

The main motivation behind BCT, as the name implies, is preserving the breast while maximizing survival. However, if the preserved breast is cosmetically unacceptable, the patient has not truly benefited from this therapy. As a consequence, factors associated with poor cosmetic outcome are considered contraindications to BCT. An unacceptable cosmetic result may occur in women with small breasts who undergo complete resection of a large tumor. In addition, women with very large breasts may have increased fibrosis because it is technically difficult to deliver a homogenous dose of radiation in these patients. Surgical treatment factors associated with poor cosmetic outcome include large volume of resection, subareolar resection, and poor scar orientation. Radiation treatment factors that may affect cosmetic outcome include fraction size, total dose, type of radiation, and concurrent chemoradiation.[3–9] For these reasons, optimal surgical and radiation techniques must be used.

Another category of contraindications to BCT addresses factors associated with a high rate of complications. These complications may also affect cosmetic outcome. Previous radiation to the breast is considered a contraindication.[10] Some evidence suggests, however, that in certain cases additional limited radiation may be possible.[11,12] Another contraindication in this category is the presence of collagen vascular diseases (connective tissue diseases) such as systemic lupus erythematosus or scleroderma.[13–15] BCT in the setting of connective tissue disorders or previous radiation may result in breast fibrosis or tissue necrosis. The evidence of increased toxicity associated with collagen vascular disease varies, however. As a consequence, collagen vascular diseases are sometimes referred to as relative contraindications. Finally, due to fear of complications, pregnancy is also included in this category. Although studies have shown that the theoretical exposure to the fetus during breast irradiation would be minimal, pregnancy is still considered an absolute contraindication to such therapy.[16,17] A pregnant woman may have a lumpectomy and receive chemotherapy, if required, until she delivers; after delivery, she may then receive breast irradiation.

The third and final category of contraindications specifically addresses in-breast recurrence risk. When the risk of in-breast recurrences is greater than 30% to 40% at 5 years, perhaps the patient is not well served by BCT and may be better served by mastectomy. Factors associated with a high rate of recurrence include positive or close margins, multiple sites of disease involving more than one quadrant (multicentric disease), lymphovascular invasion (LVI), and invasive disease with an extensive ductal carcinoma in situ (DCIS) component.[2,18–20] Factors not uniformly shown to be associated with an increased rate of in-breast failure include estrogen receptor (ER) status, histologic grade, nodal status, and HER2/neu overexpression. Patients who are *BRCA1*- or *BRCA2*-positive do not have a higher rate of local failures and, therefore, are candidates for BCT.[21,22]

Of special note is young age. Women younger than age 35 to 40 years have an increased rate of local failure when compared to their older counterparts for reasons that are not exactly clear.[20,23,24] Nonetheless, when BCT is compared to mastectomy in younger patients, local control and survival rates are similar. Therefore, young age alone is not a contraindication to BCT.

Fortunately, the majority of women are candidates for BCT. The most common candidate for BCT is a woman with a single tumor smaller than 4 cm that has been completely resected and with negative margins.

Invasive Breast Cancer Treatment Outcome

Several prospective randomized trials have shown that the rate of local failure (LF) after lumpectomy alone may be as high as 30% to 40% at 5 years; however, if radiation is administered, the LF rate is reduced to approximately 10% at 5 years.[1] Although 75% of all LFs occur within the first 5 years after treatment, late local recurrences have been reported at 15 to 20 years after treatment.

Until recently, most evidence supported equivalent survival between modified radical mastectomy (MRM) and BCT groups. However, there is now clear evidence, obtained via large meta-analyses, of a survival benefit with adjuvant radiation in BCT. The Early Breast Cancer Trialists' Collaborative Group (EBCTCG) evaluated seven prospective randomized trials comparing breast-conserving surgery (BCS) with and without adjuvant radiation. In their 2005 update with 15 years of follow-up, the authors showed a statistically significant absolute 5% survival benefit in women who received radiation.[1] Vinh-Hung et al. showed a survival benefit of 8.5% in their meta-analysis in favor of adjuvant radiation.[25] Thus it is now clear that radiation not only reduces local recurrence after BCS, but also provides a real survival benefit.

NONINVASIVE BREAST CANCER

Breast-Conserving Therapy

The increased use of screening has led to a shift in the diagnosis of breast cancer from later to earlier stages of the disease. Approximately 20% of all new breast cancer diagnoses involve DCIS. Unlike with invasive breast cancer, no randomized trials have as yet compared BCT to mastectomy. The closest was a trial by error. When reviewing the path for patients participating in the National Surgical Adjuvant Breast Project (NSABP) B-06 trial who were randomized to lumpectomy alone, lumpectomy and radiation, or mastectomy, it was discovered that some of the patients enrolled in this invasive breast cancer trial actually had only DCIS.[26] The patients with DCIS were evenly distributed among the three treatment arms. At a median follow-up of 39 months, the local failure rates in the lumpectomy patients with and without adjuvant radiation were 7% and 23%, respectively. There was no difference in survival among patients who had undergone lumpectomy alone, lumpectomy and radiation, or mastectomy, respectively.

Two large randomized, prospective trials have compared lumpectomy alone to lumpectomy and radiation in patients with DCIS: NSABP B-17 and European Organisation for Research and Treatment of Cancer (EORTC) 10853.[27,28] In both trials, the rate of local recurrence was reduced by approximately 50% with adjuvant radiation. In B-17, the rates of recurrence at eight years in the lumpectomy-alone and lumpectomy-plus-radiation arms were 31% and 13%, respectively. In the EORTC trial with 10-year follow-up, the local failure rates were 26% and 15%, respectively, with the corresponding treatments. Factors associated with an increased rate of local failure included young age, solid and cribriform subtypes, positive margins, symptomatic detection of DCIS, and lack of radiation.[29]

Many researchers have attempted to identify patients with DCIS who may be healed with conservative surgery alone. Probably the most well-known decision tool for this purpose is the Van Nuys Prognostic Index (VNPI), which was first published by Silverstein et al.[30] This prognostic index divides patients into three risk groups from which decisions about radiation or mastectomy may be made. Unfortunately, although very attractive, the VNPI has not been reliably verified in other studies. De Mascarel et al. were not able to reproduce the VNPI results,[31] nor were Fisher et al. able to do so when this classification system was applied to patients treated on B-17.[29] Nonetheless, there is such great interest in defining a group of patients who could be treated with surgery alone that two large U.S. trials have addressed this issue. Eastern Cooperative Oncology Group (ECOG) registry trial E5194 is following patients with DCIS who did not receive radiation after lumpectomy. The other trial sponsored by the Radiation Therapy Oncology Group, RTOG 98-04, is randomizing women with DCIS to radiation or not, with or without adjuvant tamoxifen. The role of tamoxifen in the management of DCIS is discussed elsewhere in this book.

While the results of RTOG 98-04 are not yet available, preliminary results of E5194 have been presented.[32] The latter study enrolled 711 patients. To qualify for inclusion, patients had to have a low/intermediate-grade DCIS (2.5 cm or smaller) or high-grade DCIS (1.0 cm or smaller). All patients had to have a resected surgical margin of 3.0 cm or larger. After 5.4 years median follow-up, the rates of ipsilateral breast events in patients with low/intermediate-grade and high-grade DCIS were 6.1% and 14.8%, respectively. The authors concluded that carefully selected patients with low/intermediate-grade DCIS who do not receive radiation have an acceptably low rate of ipsilateral breast events. However, they also recognized that these results are preliminary and stated that further follow-up is necessary.

BCT Radiation Techniques

A typical radiation treatment course after lumpectomy lasts 5 to 7 weeks. During the first 5 weeks or so, the entire breast is treated via tangential beams to a dose necessary to kill microscopic subclinical disease (4500 to 5000 cGy). This is followed by treatment to the lumpectomy bed alone for 1 to 2 weeks with an additional 1000 to 2000 cGy (also known as "boost" therapy). While the benefit of a boost is established in invasive breast cancer, the role of a boost in the treatment of DCIS is less certain.

Often it is necessary to treat the nodal groups in patients who have had BCS for invasive breast cancer. The indications for nodal irradiation are discussed in the postmastectomy radiation therapy section of this chapter. Because the risk of nodal metastases in DCIS is less than 1% to 2%, there is no routine surgical evaluation of the axilla or regional node irradiation for this diagnosis.

Tattoos and nonpermanent marks are placed on the skin of the chest to aid in daily setup for radiation treatments. Should the patient need radiation to the opposite breast in the future, these tattoos serve as permanent marks from which past treatment fields may be reproduced and then avoided. Given this fact, patients should consider this potential future purpose of the tattoos before deciding to have them removed.

Postmastectomy Radiation

Some of the earliest randomized prospective trials in oncology addressed the role of radiation after mastectomy for breast cancer. These early trials clearly showed a local control benefit with postmastectomy radiation (PMXRT). Unfortunately, evidence of a survival benefit was lacking. Meta-analysis of these early trials showed a survival detriment with PMXRT, with most of these deaths being of cardiac etiology.[33] As a consequence, PMXRT was reserved for the most advanced cases.

In 1997, the results of three randomized prospective trials of PMXRT were published. All three trials showed not only a local control benefit with PMXRT, like that seen in many of the earlier trials, but also a statistically significant survival benefit. These trials, in contrast to their predecessors, benefited from modern standardized radiation therapy techniques as well as modern chemotherapy.[34,35]

Many criticized these trials on both systemic and local therapeutic grounds. The criticisms concerning systemic therapy centered on the use of the cyclophosphamide/methotrexate/5-fluorouracil (CMF) regimen in two of the trials and the use of tamoxifen in the third study. One might argue that the results of these PMXRT trials are not applicable to the current breast cancer patient for two reasons: (1) CMF is not the most common first-line chemotherapy regimen in breast cancer and (2) tamoxifen, which was prescribed for only 1 year in the study, is usually prescribed for 5 years.

While most agree that patients with four or more positive nodes should receive post-mastectomy radiation, there is a disagreement with respect to patients with one to three positive nodes. The high rate of LF in patients who did not receive radiation therapy is at the core of the remaining criticisms. In all three trials, there was an unusually high rate (30% to 33%) of local regional failure in the patients with one to three positive lymph nodes who did not receive radiation. This rate stands in contrast to the local regional failure rate of 13% in patients with one to three positive nodes observed in a review of many prospective U.S. trials.[36] Some have argued that inadequate surgery—specifically, an inadequate axillary dissection—may be the cause of the high rate of LF in the PMXRT trials; if true, this means that the use of radiation therapy compensated for less-than-ideal surgery. An attempt to specifically address these concerns was made via a large Phase III trial that randomized women with one to three positive lymph nodes to either receive radiation or not. Unfortunately, the trial was closed prematurely when it failed to enroll an adequate number of patients.

The controversy over whether to offer PMXRT to patients with one to three positive lymph nodes may soon be ending. A retrospective study by Buchholz et al. showed a survival benefit of adjuvant radiation in women with one to three positive lymph nodes when compared to similar patients who were treated with mastectomy alone.[37] In addition, the EBCTCG presented a meta-analysis of more than 3000 women with one to three positive nodes who had been treated with mastectomy, axillary clearance, and radiation; the majority of these patients had received systemic therapy. In this study, the authors reported a statistically significant overall survival benefit in favor of adjuvant radiation.[38] These reports suggest that the distinction made between one to three positive axillary lymph nodes and four or more positive nodes in deciding whether to offer adjuvant radiation therapy should be abandoned. Consequently, it is our practice to offer PMXRT to all women with positive axillary lymph nodes.

Postmastectomy Radiation Technique

Because all three randomized trials showing a survival benefit of PMXRT used similar radiation fields and biologic effective doses, we recommend that similar fields and doses be utilized for PMXRT. In all three trials, the chest wall, supraclavicular, and internal mammary nodes were irradiated. The axilla was included in all trials, although it may not have received full dose. Similar fields are recommended for women with axillary node-positive disease who are also undergoing BCT.

The utility of internal mammary lymph node (IMLN) radiation often generates vigorous debate. Some claim that a recurrence in an IMLN is sufficiently rare that routine treatment of this nodal group is not warranted.[39] We disagree. There are basically three lines of evidence that we believe justify our treatment of the IMLNs.

▷ These three PMXRT trials, all of which irradiated the IMLNs, are the first to show a clear survival benefit with PMXRT.

▷ Two pathologic series, performed approximately 30 years apart and evaluating the incidence of IMLN metastases, revealed essentially the same result.[40–43] In these two series, there was a 9% to 13% risk of pathologically positive IMLNs in women with a pathologically negative axilla. However, this risk increased to 28% to 37% in patients with a pathologically positive axilla.

▷ In a report by Stemmer et al., women participating in a bone marrow transplant trial received PMXRT, which included IMLN irradiation via electrons.[44] Halfway through the trial, the researchers lost electron therapy capability and discontinued treatment of the IMLNs. With a median follow up of seven months, the authors reported a statistically significant improvement in disease-free survival (DFS) and a trend towards improved overall survival (OAS) in favor of IMLN irradiation.

Based on these lines of evidence, we conclude that IMLN irradiation should be considered for patients who are receiving adjuvant nodal irradiation axillary.

The dose of radiation is typically 4600 to 5000 cGy, delivered over a 5-week period to all fields. The delivery of a boost dose to the scar occurs at the physician's discretion. In addition, bolus or bolus-equivalent material is placed on the chest wall during treatment. The purpose of this material is to ensure that a therapeutic dose is delivered to the skin.

RADIATION TOXICITY

Breast-Conserving Therapy

Radiation therapy, although beneficial in improving both local control and survival, is not without social and physical costs. The social costs are lost time from loved ones and livelihood, whereas the physical costs may include rib, lung, nerve, and soft-tissue damage. It is important to note that toxic effects of radiation can be affected by several treatment- and patient-related factors. Treatment-related factors include type and energy of radiation, area treated, dose, fraction size, immobilization devices, and dosimetric plans.[45,46] Patient-related factors associated with increased toxicity include body mass index (BMI), concurrent chemotherapy, comorbidities (i.e., diabetes, connective tissue diseases, renal failure, smoking), and previous radiation exposure.[47]

Side effects or toxicities can be separated into two general categories: early and late. Early (or acute) toxicities occur during the course of radiation; late toxicities may occur 6 weeks to several years after radiation. The most common acute side effects from whole-breast radiation are fatigue and skin irritation. The severity and incidence of these side effects and all others vary greatly from patient to patient, however. The fatigue tends to be very mild such that many women are able to continue working full-time during the course of treatment. Skin irritation, or radiation dermatitis, is also fairly common. In some studies, as many as 90% of patients have developed some form of radiation dermatitis.[48]

The deep layer of the epidermis contains basal stem cells. These stem cells are responsible for maintaining the cells that make up the cornified layer of the epidermis. Radiation damages these stem cells. As a consequence, there is shedding of the cornified layer (dry desquamation). The radiation therapy may also cause capillary dilatation, increased permeability, and an inflammatory response resulting in erythema and edema. There is also hyperpigmentation from migration of the melanocytes to the surface. Radiation-induced epilation, plus loss of sweat and sebaceous glands, results in dry and pruritic skin. With continued loss of the basal cell layer, the dermis will then be exposed (moist desquamation), which may progress to frank ulceration. Healing entails reepithelialization via repopulation of the residual basal cells or migration of basal cells from neighboring areas.[49,50] Late effects of this skin damage may include decreased skin integrity, telangectasias and change in pigmentation.

A multitude of putative treatments are available. Unfortunately, very few have been proven to be more effective than the best supportive care in clinical trials. Putative therapies include washing with mild soap, use of aloe, barrier films, corticosteroids, antimicrobial creams (silver sulfadiazide), and trolamine. Two of these treatments have been studied in a prospective fashion and found to be somewhat effective. In a randomized prospective trial, *Calendula officinalis* cream was found to significantly reduce skin toxicity when compared to trolamine.[50] Trolamine has been shown to be no better than best supportive care. Hyaluronic acid cream, when compared in a randomized prospective trial to placebo, was found to significantly delay the onset of severe skin toxicity.[50] Although ensuring a reduction in skin toxicity is a laudable goal, given the lack of effective agents, one should at minimum provide supportive care including, if possible, pain relief.

Late breast-related side effects associated with whole-breast radiation may include breast shrinkage, fibrosis, edema, telangectasias, hypopigmentation/hyperpigmentation, and tenderness.[51,52] Due to their proximity to the treated breast, other organs and structures may also be affected by radiation-induced toxicities. One such toxicity is radiation pneumonitis, which is characterized by interstitial inflammation associated with a nonproductive cough and/or low-grade fever. The risk of developing radiation pneumonitis ranges from 1% to 7% and has been linked to patient- and treatment-related factors such as obesity and radiation dose and fields.[47,51,53–55] Chemotherapy may also increase the risk of developing radiation pneumonitis. A short course of corticosteroids followed by a slow taper has been used successfully at our institution to treat this condition.

With left breast/chest wall treatment, there is a risk of radiation exposure to the heart. Meta-analyses of studies using outdated radiation techniques have shown an increased rate of cardiac events in participants who received radiation compared to those who did not.[33] This increase in cardiac events did not become obvious until 15 years after therapy. With modern radiation machines and techniques, however, there is little evidence to suggest increased cardiac morbidity with radiation. For example, in the three modern PMXRT trials in which the chest wall, supraclavicular (SCV), axillary and internal mammary lymph nodes were treated, there was no statistically significant difference in cardiac morbidity.[35,56,57] As the use of systemic chemotherapy increases, especially with agents known to be cardiotoxic (e.g., anthracyclines and trastuzamab), it is necessary to remain vigilant in avoiding and assessing the potential for radiation-induced cardiac toxicity.

Lymphedema is perhaps one of the most feared late effects of radiation therapy. The definition of lymphedema varies greatly in the literature, which inherently makes comparisons between studies and reporting the true incidence extremely difficult. At our institution, we define lymphedema as a greater than 2-cm circumference difference between the affected and nonaffected arm measured at 10 cm above and below the olecranon. This is not a universally accepted definition. Some define lymphedema as a cumulative difference of more than 10 cm between these measurements, whereas others look for a difference in volume measured by water displacement when the arm is placed in a water bath.

In part as a consequence of a failure to reach a universally accepted definition of lymphedema, reported rates of this condition vary greatly. The highest rates appear to be associated with a full axillary dissection (levels I–III) combined with axillary radiation therapy.[58] Other factors associated with an increased risk of lymphedema include obesity, age, hypertension, infection, radiation fields and dose, number of nodes removed, and number of nodes containing metastatic disease.[59–63] Fortunately, rates appear to have dropped significantly with the advent of sentinel node biopsies, limited nodal dissection (levels I–II only), and judicious use of modern radiation techniques. In the PMXRT randomized trials, lymphedema was seen in only 9% to 14% of the patients.[35] The modern incidence of lymphedema is probably in the range of 10% to 20%.

There is no cure for lymphedema. Instead, intervention is motivated by the desire to palliate symptoms and reduce risk of complications. Management of lymphedema includes massage, sequential compression, and compressive garments.[64] In addition, patients are instructed to avoid infections, blood draws, and blood pressure screening in the at-risk arm. We recommend that the patient be seen by a lymphedema specialist at the earliest sign of lymphedema.

Another feared and often-mentioned potential side effect of radiation is the development of a second, nonbreast malignancy. Approximately 7% to 8% of women undergoing adjuvant radiation for breast cancer will develop a second malignancy; nevertheless, when compared to similar patients who did not undergo radiation treatment, there does not appear to be a statistically significant difference or, if one exists, it is quite small.[65,66] Although Obedian et al.[65] and Woodward et al.[66] found no overall statistically significant difference, Galper et al.[67] reported a 1% absolute increase in second, nonbreast malignancies associated with radiation therapy. Of note, however, is the apparent increase in lung cancer in women who smoke and receive radiation therapy. Galper et al. reported a 15-year risk of developing lung cancer of 0.3%, 4.7%, and 6% in women who never smoked, who stopped smoking at diagnosis of breast cancer, and who continued to smoke after completing radiation, respectively.

Other late side effects of radiation therapy with standard fractionation include brachial plexopathy (1%), spontaneous rib weakening or fracture (2% to 3%), decreased shoulder mobility (5%), and grade 2 breast fibrosis (4%).[51,53]

ALTERNATIVE THERAPIES

Partial-Breast Irradiation

Because of the physical and social costs of whole-breast irradiation mentioned previously, there has been much interest in developing ways to facilitate BCT. One such method is partial-breast irradiation (PBI). Because the vast majority of local recurrences after BCT have been in the vicinity of the original tumor, one must ask if there is really a need to treat the whole breast. Several large, randomized trials are ongoing in both North America and Europe that are seeking to answer this question.

There are generally three ways to deliver radiation to the lumpectomy bed plus margin while minimizing the dose to the remainder of the breast (PBI). The methods can be divided into two general categories: brachytherapy and teletherapy techniques. Brachytherapy is characterized as the placement of radioactive source close to, next to, or through the target organ/tissue. Teletherapy refers to treatment in which the radioactive source is located at some distance from the target organ/tissue. The benefit of brachytherapy is that the radiation dose decreases rapidly with increasing distance from the source; therefore, it is uniquely qualified to treat small areas with high doses yet spare the surrounding tissue.

Brachytherapy may be delivered via interstitial or intracavitary techniques.[68–70] The interstitial technique consists of placing hollow needles through the breast and lumpectomy bed in multiple layers. Then, at some later time, radioactive sources are placed in those needles to treat the lumpectomy bed. The intracavitary brachytherapy technique uses a balloon, which is placed in the lumpectomy bed at the time of surgery. The balloon is inflated to approximate the walls of the cavity. A source is then placed in the center of the balloon to deliver radiation to the walls of the lumpectomy bed.

The remaining partial-breast techniques involve delivery of radiation via an external source (also known as teletherapy). Teletherapy PBI is delivered either intraoperatively or postoperatively. The intraoperative technique delivers one large dose of radiation to the exposed lumpectomy bed, either with photons or with electrons.[71–73] The postoperative technique uses three-dimensional conformal radiation therapy or intensity-modulated radiation therapy (IMRT) to deliver radiation to the lumpectomy bed plus margin.[74] The duration of postoperative PBI may range from as short as 5 days of twice-daily treatment to 15 once-daily fractions.

All of the PBI techniques described concentrate on decreasing the radiation portion of therapy. However, if one considers the entire adjuvant course of therapy for many women, decreasing only the radiation is little consolation when they are facing several months of systemic therapy. In hopes of facilitating the entire course of adjuvant breast cancer therapy, researchers at Johns Hopkins are combining PBI with concurrent dose-dense chemotherapy (PBICC).[75] A typical course of every 3-week chemotherapy followed by adjuvant radiation can range from 5 to 7 months or longer. With PBICC, the complete course of chemotherapy and radiation could be reduced to just 2 to 4 months. Although PBI and PBICC appear to be attractive options, one must remember that both are still experimental therapeutic techniques and regimens. Trials rigorously comparing PBI to standard whole-breast radiation are in progress. Until long-term follow-up is available, PBI and PBICC should not be offered outside of clinical studies.

Lumpectomy Alone

Several studies have attempted to identify a subset of breast cancer patients for whom radiation is not necessary. Despite many attempts, all of these studies have shown that radiation reduced the rate of local failure when compared to limited surgery alone. However, recent studies suggest that certain elderly women may safely consider forgoing radiation. In a trial carried out by Hughes et al., women older than age 70 were randomized to receive adjuvant radiation after lumpectomy for ER-positive tumors smaller than 2 cm.[76] Nodal status was not evaluated in all patients. All patients received tamoxifen. With 5 years of follow-up, these authors reported a statistically significant difference in local failure in favor of radiation, 1% versus 4%. These authors argue that the absolute difference is so small that radiation could be safely avoided in this group.[76] Fyles et al. reported a similarly designed trial that evaluated the efficacy of adjuvant radiation in women older than 50 years of age. In this trial, which lasted a median of 5.6 years, the rate of local failure was 0.6% and 7.7% in those who did and did not receive adjuvant radiation, respectively.[77] In both studies, a several-fold increase in local control with radiation was observed. Although this approach appears promising, longer follow-up is needed. Currently, this option may be best considered for the elderly woman with multiple comorbidities whose life expectancy is relatively short.

CONCLUSION

Radiation therapy is integral to the management of both invasive and noninvasive breast cancer. The details of delivery and patient selection are complicated processes that require a subspecialist's knowledge to fully grasp. Therefore, it behooves patients and surgeons to involve radiation oncologists as early as possible in local therapy decisions. This truly multidisciplinary approach will ensure that the patient has a chance at the best possible outcome—cure.

⟿ **Frequently Asked Questions**

1. *My patient can't decide if she wants radiation or is willing to go through with the therapy. How long after her surgery can she do radiation for DCIS and have it still be considered "effective" and appropriate to do?*

   Studies suggest that radiation can be delayed for 10 weeks or longer without necessarily being associated with a decrease in control for invasive breast cancer. It is probably safe to extrapolate these results to patients with DCIS.

2. *Under what circumstances might a patient receive radiation therapy and chemotherapy at the same time?*

   Radiation therapy and chemotherapy have been done simultaneously in the past safely, but this decision depends on which chemotherapy agents are used. There are recent reports suggesting that treatment with CMF and concurrent radiation is tolerable. Concurrent doxorubicin/cyclophosphamide (AC) and whole-breast radiation is associated with prohibitive toxicity.

3. *How is the timing of starting hormonal therapy in relationship to the patient having or completing radiation therapy determined?*

   Hormonal therapy can be started at any time.

REFERENCES

1. Clarke M, Collins R, Darby S, et al. Effects of radiotherapy and of differences in the extent of surgery for early breast cancer on local recurrence and 15-year survival: An overview of the randomised trials. Lancet 2005;366(9503):2087–2106.

2. Freedman GM, Fowble BL. Local recurrence after mastectomy or breast-conserving surgery and radiation. Oncology (Williston Park) 2000; 14(11):1561–1581; discussion 1581–1584.

3. Fujishiro S, Mitsumori M, Kokubo M, et al. Cosmetic results and complications after breast conserving therapy for early breast cancer. Breast Cancer 2000;7(1):57–63.

4. Johansen J, Overgaard J, Rose C, et al. Cosmetic outcome and breast morbidity in breast-conserving treatment: Results from the Danish

DBCG-82TM national randomized trial in breast cancer. Acta Oncol 2002:41(4):369–380.

5. Lilla C, Ambrosone CB, Kropp S, et al. Predictive factors for late normal tissue complications following radiotherapy for breast cancer. Breast Cancer Res Treat 2007 (in press).

6. Moro G, Stasi M, Borca VC. Does concomitant chemoradiotherapy influence cosmetic outcome in conservative treatment of breast cancer? Tumori 1997;83(4):743–747.

7. Palazzi M, Tomatis S, Valli MC, et al. Impact of radiotherapy technique on the outcome of early breast cancer treated with conservative surgery: A multicenter observational study on 1,176 patients. Int J Radiat Oncol Biol Phys 2006;65(5):1361–1367.

8. Sarin R, Dinshaw KA, Shrivastava SK, et al. Therapeutic factors influencing the cosmetic outcome and late complications in the conservative management of early breast cancer. Int J Radiat Oncol Biol Phys 1993; 27(2):285–292.

9. Taylor ME, Perez CA, Halverson KJ, et al. Factors influencing cosmetic results after conservation therapy for breast cancer. Int J Radiat Oncol Biol Phys 1995;31(4):753–764.

10. Wolden SL, Hancock SL, Carlson RW, et al. Management of breast cancer after Hodgkin's disease. J Clin Oncol 2000;18(4):765–772.

11. Deutsch M. Repeat high-dose external beam irradiation for in-breast tumor recurrence after previous lumpectomy and whole breast irradiation. Int J Radiat Oncol Biol Phys 2002;53(3):687–691.

12. Niehoff P, Dietrich J, Ostertag H, et al. High-dose-rate (HDR) or pulsed-dose-rate (PDR) perioperative interstitial intensity-modulated brachytherapy (IMBT) for local recurrences of previously irradiated breast or thoracic wall following breast cancer. Strahlenther Onkol 2006;182(2): 102–107.

13. Chen AM, Obedian E, Haffty BG. Breast-conserving therapy in the setting of collagen vascular disease. Cancer J 2001;(6):480–491.

14. De Naeyer B, De Meerleer G, Braems S, et al. Collagen vascular diseases and radiation therapy: A critical review. Int J Radiat Oncol Biol Phys 1999;44(5):975–980.

15. Ross JG, Hussey DH, Mayr NA, et al. Acute and late reactions to radiation therapy in patients with collagen vascular diseases. Cancer 1993; 71(11):3744–3752.

16. Bradley B, Fleck A, Osei EK. Normalized data for the estimation of fetal radiation dose from radiotherapy of the breast. Br J Radiol 2006;79(946): 818–827.

17. Mazonakis M, Varveris H, Damilakis J, et al. Radiation dose to conceptus resulting from tangential breast irradiation. Int J Radiat Oncol Biol Phys 2003;55(2):386–391.

18. Fowble B. Ipsilateral breast tumor recurrence following breast-conserving surgery for early-stage invasive cancer. Acta Oncol 1999;38(suppl 13): 9–17.

19. Freedman GM, Hanlon AL, Fowble BL, et al. Recursive partitioning identifies patients at high and low risk for ipsilateral tumor recurrence after breast-conserving surgery and radiation. J Clin Oncol 2002;20(19): 4015–4021.

20. Neri A, Marrelli D, Rossi S, et al. Breast cancer local recurrence: Risk factors and prognostic relevance of early time to recurrence. World J Surg 2007;31(1):36–45.

21. Kirova YM, Stoppa-Lyonnet D, Savignoni A, et al. Risk of breast cancer recurrence and contralateral breast cancer in relation to *BRCA1* and *BRCA2* mutation status following breast-conserving surgery and radiotherapy. Eur J Cancer 2005;41(15):2304–2311.

22. Harris EE, Hwang WT, Lee EA, et al. The impact of HER-2 status on local recurrence in women with stage I–II breast cancer treated with breast-conserving therapy. Breast J 2006;12(5):431–436.

23. Komoike Y, Akiyama F, Iino Y, et al. Ipsilateral breast tumor recurrence (IBTR) after breast-conserving treatment for early breast cancer: Risk factors and impact on distant metastases. Cancer 2006;106(1):35–41.

24. Zhou P, Gautam S, Recht A. Factors affecting outcome for young women with early-stage invasive breast cancer treated with breast-conserving therapy. Breast Cancer Res Treat 2007;101(1):51–57.

25. Vinh-Hung V, Verschraegen C. Breast-conserving surgery with or without radiotherapy: Pooled-analysis for risks of ipsilateral breast tumor recurrence and mortality. J Natl Cancer Inst 2004;96(2):115–121.

26. Fisher ER, Sass R, Fisher B, et al. Pathologic findings from the National Surgical Adjuvant Breast Project (protocol 6). I. Intraductal carcinoma (DCIS). Cancer 1986;57(2):197–208.

27. Fisher B, Dignam J, Wolmark N, et al. Lumpectomy and radiation therapy for the treatment of intraductal breast cancer: Findings from National Surgical Adjuvant Breast and Bowel Project B-17. J Clin Oncol 1998;16(2):441–452.

28. EORTC Breast Cancer Cooperative Group, EORTC Radiotherapy Group, Bijker N, et al. Breast-conserving treatment with or without radiotherapy in ductal carcinoma-in-situ: Ten-year results of European Organisation for Research and Treatment of Cancer randomized Phase III

trial 10853—a study by the EORTC Breast Cancer Cooperative Group and EORTC Radiotherapy Group. J Clin Oncol 2006;24(21):3381–3387.

29. Fisher ER, Dignam J, Tan-Chiu E, et al. Pathologic findings from the National Surgical Adjuvant Breast Project (NSABP) eight-year update of protocol B-17: Intraductal carcinoma. Cancer 1999;86(3):429–438.

30. Silverstein MJ, Poller DN, Waisman JR, et al. Prognostic classification of breast ductal carcinoma-in-situ. Lancet 1995;345(8958):1154–1157.

31. De Mascarel I, Bonichon F, MacGrogan G, et al. Application of the Van Nuys Prognostic Index in a retrospective series of 367 ductal carcinomas in situ of the breast examined by serial macroscopic sectioning: Practical considerations. Breast Cancer Res Treat 2000;61(2):151–159.

32. Hughes L, Wang M, Page D, et al. Five year results of intergroup study E5194: Local excision alone for selected patients with DCIS of the breast. San Antonio Breast Cancer Symposium, December 14–17, 2006.

33. Cuzick J, Stewart H, Rutqvist L, et al. Cause-specific mortality in long-term survivors of breast cancer who participated in trials of radiotherapy. J Clin Oncol 1994;12(3):447–453.

34. Overgaard M. Overview of randomized trials in high risk breast cancer patients treated with adjuvant systemic therapy with or without post-mastectomy irradiation. Semin Radiat Oncol 1999;9(3):292–299.

35. Ragaz J, Olivotto IA, Spinelli JJ, et al. Locoregional radiation therapy in patients with high-risk breast cancer receiving adjuvant chemotherapy: 20-year results of the British Columbia randomized trial. J Natl Cancer Inst 2005;97(2):116–126.

36. Recht A, Gray R, Davidson NE, et al. Locoregional failure 10 years after mastectomy and adjuvant chemotherapy with or without tamoxifen without irradiation: Experience of the Eastern Cooperative Oncology Group. J Clin Oncol 1999;17(6):1689–1700.

37. Buchholz TA, Woodward WA, Duan Z, et al. Radiation use and long-term survival in breast cancer patients with T1, T2 primary tumors and 1–3 positive axillary lymph nodes. Int J Radiat Oncol Biol Phys 2006; 66(3):S5.

38. McGale P, Darby S, Taylor C, et al. The 2006 worldwide overview of the effects of local treatments for early breast cancer on long term outcome. Int J Radiat Oncol Biol Phys 2006;66(3):S2.

39. Fowble B, Hanlon A, Freedman G, et al. Internal mammary node irradiation neither decreases distant metastases nor improves survival in stage I and II breast cancer. Int J Radiat Oncol Biol Phys 2000;47(4):883–894.

40. Yu J, Li G, Li J, et al. The pattern of lymphatic metastasis of breast cancer and its influence on the delineation of radiation fields. Int J Radiat Oncol Biol 2005;Phys 61(3):874–878.

41. Veronesi U, Valagussa P. Inefficacy of internal mammary nodes dissection in breast cancer surgery. Cancer 1981;47(1):170–175.

42. Veronesi U, Cascinelli N, Greco M, et al. Prognosis of breast cancer patients after mastectomy and dissection of internal mammary nodes. Ann Surg 1985;202(6):702–707.

43. Veronesi U, Cascinelli N, Bufalino R, et al. Risk of internal mammary lymph node metastases and its relevance on prognosis of breast cancer patients. Ann Surg 1983;198(6):681–684.

44. Stemmer SM, Rizel S, Hardan I, et al. The role of irradiation of the internal mammary lymph nodes in high-risk stage II to IIIA breast cancer patients after high-dose chemotherapy: A prospective sequential non-randomized study. J Clin Oncol 2003;21(14):2713–2718.

45. Altundag M, Altundag K, Cengiz M, et al. The field of radiation therapy may affect health-related quality of life in patients with operable breast cancer. J Clin Oncol 2004;22(9):1765; author reply, 1765–1766.

46. Hojris I, Andersen J, Overgaard M, et al. Late treatment-related morbidity in breast cancer patients randomized to postmastectomy radiotherapy and systemic treatment versus systemic treatment alone. Acta Oncol 2000;39(3):355–372.

47. Allen AM, Prosnitz RG, Ten Haken RK, et al. Body mass index predicts the incidence of radiation pneumonitis in breast cancer patients. Cancer J 2005;11(5):390–398.

48. Porock D, Kristjanson L. Skin reactions during radiotherapy for breast cancer: The use and impact of topical agents and dressings. Eur J Cancer Care (UK) 1999;8(3):143–153.

49. McQuestion M. Evidence-based skin care management in radiation therapy. Semin Oncol Nurs 2006;22(3):163–173.

50. Pommier P, Gomez F, Sunyach MP, et al. Phase III randomized trial of *Calendula officinalis* compared with trolamine for the prevention of acute dermatitis during irradiation for breast cancer. J Clin Oncol 2004;22(8): 1447–1453.

51. Meric F, Buchholz TA, Mirza NQ, et al. Long-term complications associated with breast-conservation surgery and radiotherapy. Ann Surg Oncol 2002;9(6):543–549.

52. Harper JL, Franklin LE, Jenrette JM, et al. Skin toxicity during breast irradiation: Pathophysiology and management. South Med J 2004;97(10): 989–993.

53. Lind PA, Wennberg B, Gagliardi G, et al. ROC curves and evaluation of radiation-induced pulmonary toxicity in breast cancer. Int J Radiat Oncol Biol Phys 2006;64(3):765–770.

54. Lind PA, Marks LB, Hardenbergh PH, et al. Technical factors associated with radiation pneumonitis after local +/− regional radiation therapy for breast cancer. Int J Radiat Oncol Biol Phys 2002;52(1):137–143.

55. Minor GI, Yashar CM, Spanos WJ Jr, et al. The relationship of radiation pneumonitis to treated lung volume in breast conservation therapy. Breast J 2006;12(1):48–52.

56. Hojris I, Andersen J, Overgaard M, et al. Late treatment-related morbidity in breast cancer patients randomized to postmastectomy radiotherapy and systemic treatment versus systemic treatment alone. Acta Oncol 2000;39(3):355–372.

57. Hojris I, Overgaard M, Christensen JJ, et al. Morbidity and mortality of ischaemic heart disease in high-risk breast-cancer patients after adjuvant postmastectomy systemic treatment with or without radiotherapy: Analysis of DBCG 82b and 82c randomised trials. Radiotherapy Committee of the Danish Breast Cancer Cooperative Group. Lancet 1999; 354(9188):1425–1430.

58. Coen JJ, Taghian AG, Kachnic LA, et al. Risk of lymphedema after regional nodal irradiation with breast conservation therapy. Int J Radiat Oncol Biol Phys 2003;55(5):1209–1215.

59. Golshan M, Martin WJ, Dowlatshahi K. Sentinel lymph node biopsy lowers the rate of lymphedema when compared with standard axillary lymph node dissection. Am Surg 2003;69(3):209–211; discussion 212.

60. Golshan M, Smith B. Prevention and management of arm lymphedema in the patient with breast cancer. J Support Oncol 2006;4(8):381–386.

61. Hinrichs CS, Watroba NL, Rezaishiraz H, et al. Lymphedema secondary to postmastectomy radiation: Incidence and risk factors. Ann Surg Oncol 2004;11(6):573–580.

62. Silberman AW, McVay C, Cohen JS, et al. Comparative morbidity of axillary lymph node dissection and the sentinel lymph node technique: Implications for patients with breast cancer. Ann Surg 2004;240(1):1–6.

63. Kocak Z, Overgaard J. Risk factors of arm lymphedema in breast cancer patients. Acta Oncol 2000;39(3):389–392.

64. Kligman L, Wong RK, Johnston M, et al. The treatment of lymphedema related to breast cancer: A systematic review and evidence summary. Support Care Cancer 2004;12(6):421–431.

65. Obedian E, Fischer DB, Haffty BG. Second malignancies after treatment of early-stage breast cancer: Lumpectomy and radiation therapy versus mastectomy. J Clin Oncol 2000;18(12):2406–2412.

66. Woodward WA, Strom EA, McNeese MD, et al. Cardiovascular death and second non-breast cancer malignancy after postmastectomy radia-

tion and doxorubicin-based chemotherapy. Int J Radiat Oncol Biol Phys 2003;57(2):327–335.

67. Galper S, Gelman R, Recht A, et al. Second nonbreast malignancies after conservative surgery and radiation therapy for early-stage breast cancer. Int J Radiat Oncol Biol Phys 2002;52(2):406–414.

68. Benitez PR, Chen PY, Vicini FA, et al. Partial breast irradiation in breast conserving therapy by way of interstitial brachytherapy. Am J Surg 2004;188(4):355–364.

69. Benitez PR, Streeter O, Vicini F, et al. Preliminary results and evaluation of MammoSite balloon brachytherapy for partial breast irradiation for pure ductal carcinoma in situ: A Phase II clinical study. Am J Surg 2006; 192(4):427–433.

70. Chen PY, Vicini FA, Benitez P, et al. Long-term cosmetic results and toxicity after accelerated partial-breast irradiation: A method of radiation delivery by interstitial brachytherapy for the treatment of early-stage breast carcinoma. Cancer 2006;106(5):991–999.

71. Orecchia R, Ciocca M, Lazzari R, et al. Intraoperative radiation therapy with electrons (ELIOT) in early-stage breast cancer. Breast 2003;12(6): 483–490.

72. Orecchia R, Luini A, Veronesi P, et al. Electron intraoperative treatment in patients with early-stage breast cancer: Data update. Expert Rev Anticancer Ther 2006;6(4):605–611.

73. Vaidya JS, Baum M, Tobias JS, et al. The novel technique of delivering targeted intraoperative radiotherapy (Targit) for early breast cancer. Eur J Surg Oncol 2002;28(4):447–454.

74. Vicini FA, Remouchamps V, Wallace M, et al. Ongoing clinical experience utilizing 3D conformal external beam radiotherapy to deliver partial-breast irradiation in patients with early-stage breast cancer treated with breast-conserving therapy. Int J Radiat Oncol Biol Phys 2003;57(5): 1247–1253.

75. Zellars R, Frassica D, Stearns V, et al. Partial breast irradiation (PBI) concurrent with adjuvant dose-dense doxorubicin and cyclophosphamide (ddAC) chemotherapy in early stage breast cancer: Preliminary safety results from a feasibility trial. Int J Radiat Oncol Biol Phys 2006;66(3):S217.

76. Hughes KS, Schnaper LA, Berry D, et al. Lumpectomy plus tamoxifen with or without irradiation in women 70 years of age or older with early breast cancer. N Engl J Med 2004;351(10):971–977.

77. Fyles AW, McCready DR, Manchul LA, et al. Tamoxifen with or without breast irradiation in women 50 years of age or older with early breast cancer. N Engl J Med 2004;351(10):963–970.

Algorithm for Hormonal Therapy

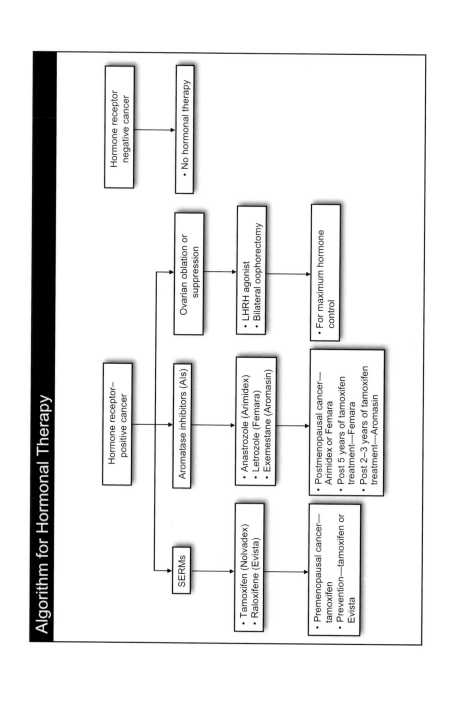

chapter

9

Hormonal Therapy

Lillie D. Shockney, RN, BS, MAS

What you need to know:

Approximately 50% of women are candidates for hormonal therapy and are advised to take it to prevent breast cancer recurrence. These women have tumors that are sensitive to estrogen [estrogen receptor positive (ER+)] or progesterone [progesterone receptor positive (PR+)] as determined by histopathologic evaluation.

Patient education is paramount for ensuring compliance with hormonal therapy. This is due in part to the need to take the drug for several years, combined with its many possible side effects, which may lead to frustration in some patients.

Each time you see your patient, you should ask her how she is doing on her hormonal therapy and reiterate this treatment's role in breast cancer prevention.

Premenopausal women are prescribed selective estrogen-receptor modulators (SERMs) and postmenopausal women are prescribed aromatase inhibitors (AIs). The only exception to this practice occurs with women who are diagnosed with ductal carcinoma in situ (DCIS). Women with DCIS, no matter what their menopausal status, are usually prescribed tamoxifen, a SERM.

The risk of uterine cancer and deep vein thrombosis (DVT), or both, from taking tamoxifen is extremely low. Nevertheless, many patients assume that their risk for these conditions is high. They need reassurance that this is not the case. Women who are usually advised not to take this drug are smokers and those with a previous history of DVT, transient ischemic attack (TIA), or stroke.

AIs can result in bone loss, so bone density tests are important for monitoring the bone health of patients who take these agents. You may to prescribe bisphosphonates in such cases.

Because of estrogen depletion, cholesterol levels should also be monitored on a routine basis.

Patients should not take any form of hormone replacement therapy (HRT) if they are diagnosed with breast cancer. If a patient is taking HRT and receives this diagnosis, she needs to be weaned off the HRT soon after her diagnosis and must remain off of this medication, even if her tumor was hormone receptor negative.

Educate your premenopausal patient about the importance of continuing some effective means of birth control even if she is not menstruating during hormonal therapy.

If your patient has limited finances, most drug companies provide a discounted program for obtaining the hormonal therapy agents they manufacture.

Ovarian ablation or suppression is used for *BRCA1*- or *BRCA2*-positive patients to prevent breast cancer as well as ovarian cancer. It is also used as a means of providing maximum hormonal control.

Hormonal therapy (SERMs) may also be prescribed for women who are at a high risk of developing breast cancer—those with a significant family history or who are positive for the *BRCA1* or *BRCA2* gene—and have elected to not have preventive mastectomy surgery.

What your patient needs to know:

Women who have tumors that are hormone receptor positive are commonly advised to take hormonal therapy. Hormonal therapy is not to be confused with HRT. In fact, the patient should actually think of the two as being polar opposites.

Approximately 50% of women who are diagnosed with breast cancer will be advised to take hormonal therapy. Hormonal therapy is also prescribed to high-risk women as a means of preventing breast cancer.

It is extremely important to take the medication as prescribed. If the patient is experiencing side effects that are affecting her quality of life, she needs to notify her oncologist and discuss methods to reduce these side effects with the goal of maintaining her on hormonal therapy.

There are two categories of hormonal therapy: SERMs and AIs. SERMs are usually prescribed for premenopausal women and AIs for postmenopausal women.

Even if a woman no longer has her ovaries, her body can still manufacture estrogen through her adrenal glands. She also stores estrogen in her body fat.

Women who have been diagnosed with breast cancer should not take any form of HRT. This group includes women whose breast cancer was hormone receptor negative.

Menopausal symptoms are the most common symptoms reported with HRT. If these symptoms are severe, doctors can recommend drugs and methods to reduce these side effects.

Patients have a tendency to want to jump from one form of hormonal therapy to another in hopes of experiencing fewer and less severe side effects. No data have been collected on the effect of switching therapies in this way from the perspective of risk reduction. Women commonly ask for the hormonal therapy with the least side effects rather than asking which hormonal therapy is the most effective for the particular clinical situation.

Women may experience other medical problems as a result of taking hormonal therapy, including bone loss when taking an AI. Regular exercise and calcium intake are recommended for patients who take AIs. In some cases, patients may be advised to take a prescription bone-building agent. Cholesterol elevation may also be an issue when taking AIs, so it important for the patient to watch her fat intake and for her doctor to monitor her blood levels on a routine basis.

Most women assume that tamoxifen will cause uterine cancer and/or stroke. The incidence of these serious complications is actually very low. Women taking this drug should not smoke, however.

Hormonal therapy is taken for several years. Thus the patient needs to make a commitment to herself and to her doctors that she will be compliant in taking the medication daily and at the recommended dose.

$\approx$ $\approx$ $\approx$

INTRODUCTION

Nonadherence with prescribed medication is an age-old problem. Despite the ability of medicines to prevent, relieve, and even cure many types of illness, people often do not take them as prescribed.[1] The potential to improve health outcomes through better compliance with therapy represents an enormous opportunity in terms of both reducing patient burden and decreasing the cost of disease management.

Studies that have been conducted by various pharmaceutical companies based on interviews with oncologists have found that most doctors believe their patients are compliant in taking their medications as prescribed.[2] The data from the patients, however, tell a different story. Awareness of this problem may be the first critical step in improving adherence to maintain optimal health. Despite the fact that breast cancer is a serious disease, patients do not always take their medications as prescribed. As former surgeon General C. Everett Koop stated, "Drugs don't work in patients who don't take them."[3]

A large percentage (50%) of breast cancer patients are advised to take hormonal therapy after completing their breast cancer treatment comprising surgery, chemotherapy, and/or radiation therapy. Today, hormonal therapy commonly is prescribed for many consecutive years—even as long as a decade. During this post-treatment phase, patients are seen less often by their oncology health care providers, but it is hoped that they will periodically keep their primary care provider (PCP), gynecologist, and other health care practitioners involved in maintaining their general health and well-being. This makes your role as a health care provider for these patients increasingly important, as you will have the opportunity to promote compliance with hormonal therapy during these patient encounters. Levels of patient compliance with medications are not definitively known, even though compliance with hormonal therapy may influence its effectiveness as a means of breast cancer prevention.

The depth and content of patient education given to breast cancer survivors about the purpose of taking hormonal therapy, importance of compliance with the dose and frequency, and management of potential side effects vary among providers. Patients may not voluntarily tell their health care providers that they are not taking their medications as prescribed. This lack of compliance may be due to not understanding the importance of the drug regimen, unwillingness to cope with side effects that affect quality of life for a long period, or even embarrassment about reporting this information (i.e., sexual side effects, menopausal symptoms, lack of financial resources to purchase the medication). Clinical studies rely on, and to some degree assume, patient compliance when measuring efficacy of the drug therapy; however, compliance with self-drug administration is not one of the elements measured and assessed as part of most hormonal therapy outcomes studies.

This chapter begins with an overview of hormonal therapy and then discusses the potential side effects that can cause patients to not comply with the recommended medication regimen. The chapter also provides information about ways to reduce the side effects associated with hormonal therapy and suggests when to consider recommending that a patient contact her oncologist to discuss the hormonal therapy plan.

TYPES OF HORMONAL THERAPY

There are two categories of hormonal therapy: selective estrogen-receptor modulators (SERMs) and aromatase inhibitors (AIs). In recent years, results of studies have been published—with still more research currently under way—demonstrating the benefit of these medications in preventing recurrence of disease.

Selective Estrogen-Receptor Modulators

SERMs are prescribed to treat both premenopausal women and postmenopausal women who have noninvasive early or advanced disease (i.e., DCIS). These drugs are also approved for women who are considered to be at high risk for breast cancer even though they lack a personal history of the disease.

SERMs act on some parts of the body (such as bones) much like estrogen does and help prevent bone loss as a woman ages. They do not have estrogen-like effects on other parts of the body, however. This class of drugs works by binding (attaching) to estrogen receptors and selectively modulating the effects of estrogen in different body tissues. Because not all estrogen receptors are the same, these differences allow SERMs to have one effect in one kind of tissue and a different effect in another kind of tissue.

Tamoxifen (Nolvadex), a synthetic drug used in breast cancer prevention and treatment, was the first SERM developed and has the longest track record for use as hormonal therapy for breast cancer. It was considered the gold standard for breast cancer treatment for more than 20 years. This drug blocks the effects of estrogen on the breast and has been shown to reduce the risk of cancer recurrence as well as to prevent cancer from developing in the other (contralateral) breast. Side effects of tamoxifen include an increased risk of certain visual disturbances, fatal pulmonary embolism, and cancer of both the endometrium and the body of the uterus. The antiestrogenic effects of tamoxifen on breast cells appear to reverse after 5 years; the drug may then become cancer-promoting, for reasons that are not clear. Tamoxifen has been proven to reduce the risk of breast cancer by 47%.[4]

Raloxifene (Evista) was the second synthetic SERM to reach the market, and it is similar in some ways to tamoxifen. It is currently prescribed to protect women against osteoporosis and heart disease without increasing their risk for breast cancer. However, it does not protect bones as well as estrogen does. The results of the Study of Tamoxifen and Raloxifene Trial (STAR) have confirmed that raloxifene is as effective as tamoxifen in breast cancer prevention and may be associated with slightly fewer side effects that are worrisome to some patients, potentially resulting in a higher level of compliance with the therapy.

Other SERMs are currently being developed. Ideally, a SERM would have all the benefits of estrogen but none of the risks. No SERM is as yet available in the United States that meets those criteria, but research is under way with that goal in mind.

Common side effects of tamoxifen include hot flashes, vaginal discharge or bleeding, and menstrual irregularities. Some women also experience hair loss or skin rashes when taking this drug.

Although the complication is uncommon (less than 1% incidence), women who take tamoxifen are at increased risk of developing blood clots in their lungs and legs. These women also have a small risk of developing two different types of uterine cancer. If a patient is taking tamoxifen and experiences any sudden chest pain, shortness of breath, coughing up blood, pain or swelling in her legs, or vaginal bleeding, she should seek medical help immediately. Women taking tamoxifen should not smoke, because this behavior increases their risk of DVT and/or stroke.

Aromatase Inhibitors

AIs reduce the levels of estrogen in the body. Anastrozole (Arimidex), letrozole (Femara), and exemestane (Aromasin) are three such synthetic hormones approved by the U.S. Food and Drug Administration (FDA) for treating advanced breast cancer. Both anastrozole and letrozole have also received FDA approval for use as adjuvant therapy in early-stage breast cancer. All three of these agents are very potent drugs and can produce a marked reduction in estrogen levels.

The main source of estrogen for premenopausal women is the ovaries. When women enter menopause, their ovaries stop producing estrogen, but estrogen levels do not drop off completely. Estrogen is still present from another process in the body—the conversion of a substance from women's adrenal glands into estrogen. Specifically, this substance, androstenedione, circulates through the body to tissues such as muscle, fat, and even breast cancers themselves, where it is converted to estrogen.

The conversion of androstenedione to estrogen is driven by an enzyme called aromatase; AIs stop this conversion process. These agents differ from tamoxifen in that they actually reduce the amount of estrogen in the body. Tamoxifen, by contrast, blocks the effects of estrogen in the body by competing with estrogen for the estrogen receptor—the receptor to which estrogen binds so as to exert its effect.

Side effects associated with AIs are generally mild. In recent clinical trials with these agents, women reported hot flashes, joint pain, and muscle aches as the most bothersome side effects.

However, a major concern with AIs is the fact that they lower the body's estrogen level, which may put the patient at a higher risk for osteoporosis. If your patient is taking an AI in the adjuvant (or any other) setting, be aware of the potential for osteoporosis and the need to monitor her bone mineral density.

Lower estrogen levels in the body also affect blood lipid levels. For this reason, some doctors are concerned that AIs might increase the risk of heart problems or cardiovascular disease.

Because there are more than 30 years of research and experience with tamoxifen but a relatively brief period of experience with AIs, other side effects associated with AIs might potentially be discovered that will warrant further investigation.

STUDY RESULTS

The Arimidex/Tamoxifen, Alone or in Combination (ATAC) trial compared tamoxifen with anastrozole as the treatment given after the removal of breast cancer. This large clinical trial evaluated the use of anastrozole as adjuvant therapy for 5 years in postmenopausal women with localized hormone-receptor-positive breast cancer. In this study, the investigators found that women who were taking anastrozole were less likely to experience a breast cancer recurrence than were the women taking tamoxifen.

This study raised an important point: the need to confirm that a woman is postmenopausal by performing blood tests rather than by relying solely on whether she has been menstruating, because chemotherapy often results in a discontinuation in menses during and sometimes for several months after treatment. The patient's hormone levels, however, may signal that she still is premenopausal or peri-menopausal.

The FDA has approved the use anastrozole as an adjuvant therapy option only for postmenopausal women. The results from the ATAC trial suggest that the best treatment option for postmenopausal women with hormone-receptor-positive breast cancer is to bypass tamoxifen and start out immediately with 5 years of anastrozole as adjuvant therapy.

A second clinical trial looked into a possible next step after tamoxifen therapy. Researchers evaluated the use of letrozole (another AI) after 5 years of tamoxifen use in postmenopausal women who had been treated for breast cancer. Most experts believe that 5 years of tamoxifen treatment for early breast cancer is the optimal duration; tamoxifen therapy that last for more than 5 years does not improve outcomes and, in fact, may be harmful. Indeed, increased rates of the serious complications of uterine cancer and DVT have been reported with increased duration of tamoxifen therapy.[5]

Study results have shown that letrozole, when given after tamoxifen, reduces the risk of breast cancer recurrence by almost half. Thus letrozole provides a new extended adjuvant treatment option for women who have completed 5 years of tamoxifen therapy. The decision to use letrozole will be based on a number of factors, including an estimate of the patient's remaining risk of developing breast cancer.[6]

Results from a third clinical trial indicate that, rather than the patient taking tamoxifen for 5 years, it may be better to switch her to an AI after 2 to 3 years of tamoxifen therapy. This trial, which was called the Intergroup Exemestane Study, randomized women who had already taken tamoxifen for 2 to 3 years to one of two groups: (1) a group that completed the 5-year course of tamoxifen or (2) a group that switched to exemestane (an AI) to complete a total of 5 years of hormonal treatment.

This study demonstrated that the women who switched to exemestane had almost a one-third reduction in risk of recurrence of breast cancer, compared with women who remained on tamoxifen. Cancers in the opposite (contralateral) breast were also reduced by more than half in the women who switched to exemestane. Researchers concluded that women who elect to start tamoxifen appear to benefit from switching to exemestane after 2 to 3 years, rather than waiting until they have completed the full 5-year course of tamoxifen therapy.[7]

The findings from all three of these studies apply only to women who are postmenopausal. No benefits from AIs have been shown in women who are still having menstrual periods.

A great deal of debate has focused on the role of AIs in early-stage breast cancer. In 2006, the American Society of Clinical Oncology (ASCO) convened an expert panel to examine all of the available data related to this issue. The ASCO panel recommended that optimal adjuvant hormonal therapy for postmenopausal women with receptor-positive breast cancer include an AI as initial therapy or after treatment with tamoxifen. The panel further recommended that each woman and her doctor weigh the risks and benefits of all potential therapies based on the patient's individual circumstances.

CONTROLLING SIDE EFFECTS

Antidepressant agents are sometimes used to treat menopause-related symptoms of depression or mood changes, and they have been shown to reduce hot flashes in some studies. Some antidepressants may interact in a negative way with hormonal therapy, however, reducing its potency and effectiveness. One antidepressant that is widely recommended for menopausal patients is venlafaxine (Effexor), which appears to have the least adverse effect on how hormonal therapy functions. Another antidepressant that has shown some benefit in this patient group is gabapentin (Neurontin). A study comparing various agents for control of hot flashes provided the information shown in Table 9.1 regarding centrally active hormonal hot flash therapies.[8]

Avoiding spicy foods and hot beverages also helps reduce hot flashes. Wearing cotton clothing that is breathable, and wearing layers so that the top layer can be shed if a woman is feeling too hot, have

TABLE 9.1 ᴄᴄ Agents for Potential Control of Hot Flashes

Drug Name	Dosage	Observed Reduction	Side Effects
Bellergal	2 pills/day	Slight	Increased dry mouth, dizziness
Clonidine	0.1 mg/day (transdermal)	Significant	Increased dry mouth, difficulty sleeping, constipation, drowsiness
Methyldopa	250 mg/day	Significant	Increased fatigue, weakness, dizziness, nausea
Venlafaxine	75 mg/day	Significant	Increased dry mouth, sleeplessness, decreased appetite
Paroxetine	25 mg/day	Significant	None

been reported to help as well. In addition, vitamin E and clonidine, which are typically used for high blood pressure, can help to reduce hot flashes for some women.

Although it will rarely come up in your practice, 1% of individuals diagnosed with breast cancer are men. These patients commonly have hormone-receptor-positive tumors and may, therefore, take hormonal therapy as well. They, too, may experience the same types of side effects as female patients, especially hot flashes and night sweats.

Some physicians opt to monitor the endometrial lining of the uterus (for women taking tamoxifen) by performing an annual transvaginal ultrasound. This is usually initiated when a patient presents with new vaginal bleeding or spotting. If the lining is noted to be thicker than normal, an endometrial biopsy may be obtained on an outpatient basis.

Thyroid function sometimes changes at menopause and causes depression. This problem may be relieved by appropriate thyroid hormone replacement therapy.

Drugs used to slow bone loss include bisphosphonates [such as alendronate (Fosamax)], raloxifene, and calcitonin. Monitoring of bone density before starting an AI and during treatment is important.

Cholesterol-lowering drugs called statins have been proven to help reduce the risk of heart disease and are being explored to prevent osteoporosis.

Vaginal dryness and lack of libido are common complaints of patients who are taking hormonal therapy. Recommending vaginal lubricants (and offering samples in your office if you have any available) and discussing with the patient and her partner alternative ways to visually and physically stimulate her sexual urges are encouraged. Vaginal estradiol appears to be contraindicated in postmenopausal women who are taking adjuvant AIs.[9]

As previously, patients are advised to not take any form of HRT once they have been diagnosed with breast cancer. Women who were previously taking HRT at the time of their diagnosis may experience the most discomfort in adjusting to hormonal therapy, as the latter treatment takes them 180 degrees from where their hormone levels were prior to diagnosis. If traditional vaginal lubricants do not provide the relief the patient needs, prescribing a vaginal hormonal cream may be considered; this course of action should be discussed with the patient's oncologist first, however.

Some patients may develop urogenital atrophy as a menopausal symptom. Treatment of this problem may require a referral to a gynecologist who specializes in treating genitourinary conditions. Encouraging patients to perform Kegel exercises has been shown to mitigate this problem for some women. Emptying the bladder frequently is also helpful.

Hair loss is an issue for some patients with breast cancer. As yet, no studies are available that have definitively proved whether taking any medications (such as Rogaine) can counteract this hair loss. Women who have not yet grown back their hair following chemotherapy may battle with this problem the most, because hormonal therapy appears to keep the hair from regenerating to the degree anticipated post chemotherapy.

BIRTH CONTROL

Some women assume that if they are not menstruating, they cannot conceive. It is important to reiterate to your patient that it remains critically important to practice birth control while taking SERMs because it has not been determined that she is truly postmenopausal. SERMs can produce serious congenital anomalies so they should not be used in fertile women.

PROMOTING COMPLIANCE WITH HORMONAL THERAPY

There is a lot of information on the Internet—some helpful and some not. It is common to find breast cancer patients who are actively seeking information through this easy-to-access resource and who may shy away from taking hormonal therapy owing to fears of the side effects described by other patients. Patients should be encouraged to rely on their health care team rather than an online chat room, where misinformation—rather than evidenced-based results—may be disseminated.

Factors that influence patients' compliance with therapy have been studied. These factors include prolonged administration of the medication, side effects, poor understanding of the need for the drug and its purpose, psychological issues, cost, and low motivation. A common finding has been that patients do not understand that their disease is serious enough to warrant this additional treatment.[10]

Because there is a high likelihood that patients will see you more often than they see their oncology doctors and nurses, oncologists rely on professionals like yourself to promote compliance with hormonal therapy. When you speak with your patients, please consider discussing the following issues.

> Your oncologist has prescribed hormonal therapy [drug name] for you as a way to help prevent recurrence of your breast cancer. This is a long-term therapy that you will take for several years. I want to help you if you are experiencing any issues related to taking this medication. So fill me in on how you are doing:
>
> 1. Are you taking your hormonal therapy as prescribed?
> 2. Are you experiencing any side effects that are affecting your quality of life?
> 3. Have you discussed these side effects with your prescribing oncologist and, if so, how long ago did this discussion take place?

4. Are you experiencing any sexual side effects that we can discuss today and find solutions for?

5. Do you have a prescription plan to cover the expenses of this medication?

6. I would like to talk with your medical oncologist about the side effects that you are having so that we might together decide on some remedies for you.

Because hormonal therapy requires a long-term commitment on the part of the patient, it falls into the same category as many other medications that are used to treat chronic illnesses. With all of these medications, problems with compliance may arise over time.

Here are some additional strategies to reinforce or improve adherence with hormonal therapy:

1. All health care providers involved with the patient's care should be made aware of the issues and importance of adherence to this medication regimen.

2. Monitor the patient's compliance with her medication during each office visit. If she misses an appointment, call and inquire about her compliance.

3. Identify patients who may be at higher risk for noncompliance and provide additional monitoring steps to help ensure that they are taking their medications as prescribed.

4. Encourage the patient to report side effects and work with her to manage those side effects. This step may require a call to her oncologist to obtain more information about what is safe to prescribe in the patient's particular circumstances.

5. Keep the patient informed about research results associated with hormonal therapy so that she is an informed patient. This conversation may also serve as a catalyst for the patient to discuss any issues she has about continuing to take the medication as prescribed.

6. Assess the patient's financial situation to ensure that she can afford the medications. If cost is an issue, there are financial resources available through most of the pharmaceutical companies to offset the expense of the drug. (See the Resources section at the end of this book for more information.)

OVARIAN ABLATION OR SUPPRESSION

In recent years, the role of ovarian ablation as a therapeutic modality in both the prevention and the treatment of breast cancer has resurfaced, long after its earliest use for this purpose nearly a century ago. Bilateral oophorectomy has proved effective in reducing the risk of developing breast cancer for women who are both *BRCA1* and *BRCA2* carriers. Tamoxifen reduces the risk of breast cancer for *BRCA2* carriers but not for *BRCA1* carriers.[11]

For premenopausal women with ER-positive tumors, a second option is endocrine therapy, which aims to suppress mitogenic estrogen signaling. Until recently, 5 years of tamoxifen therapy was regarded as the standard adjuvant endocrine therapy. Ovarian ablation is also effective in treating premenopausal women, and can be achieved by surgery, radiation, or the use of a luteinizing hormone-releasing hormone (LHRH) analog such as goserelin. The tamoxifen/goserelin combination provides more effective estrogen blocking than use of either drug alone. However, given that the third generation of AIs has demonstrated improved efficacy over tamoxifen in postmenopausal women with early- or advanced-stage disease, combination treatment with goserelin plus an AI may also provide optimal blocking in premenopausal women.[12]

Although ovarian ablation is an effective adjuvant therapy for primary breast cancer, little is understood about its effect on quality of life compared with the more widely used adjuvant chemotherapy. For some women, preserving ovarian function is a priority for the future, particularly if they have not yet had a family. For premenopausal patients in whom estrogen synthesis occurs primarily in the ovaries, treatment options may include ovarian ablation or suppression along with hormonal therapy. Although some studies have demonstrated that ovarian ablation results in an outcome equivalent to that achieved with chemotherapy alone, studies examining the combination therapy have not demonstrated a clear benefit with the addition of ovarian suppression to standard chemotherapy.[13]

CONCLUSION

Studies are under way at Johns Hopkins to better understand the barriers patients are experiencing that result in them choosing to not take their medication daily at the recommended dose. Some of these barriers include physical side effects experienced when taking the medication, fear of developing a serious complication caused by the medication, lack of understanding of the purpose of the medication, and financial limitations. The latter barrier can often be overcome by accessing the special programs available from the pharmaceutical companies that manufacture these medications, which are intended to help patients offset the costs of these expensive medications. (See the Resources section at the end of this book for more details.)

When a woman is initially diagnosed with breast cancer, she wants to do all that she can to rid herself of the disease and reduce her risk of recurrence. As more time goes by, and the patient is past the period when the risk of recurrence is its highest (the first 2 years), she may begin weighing the pros and cons of taking medications that are causing her unpleasant side effects against the benefit of reducing her risk. Quality of life is a priority for these women—as it should be. As health care professionals, we need to help our patients find a sense of balance in reducing the risk of recurrence while maintaining an active, enjoyable lifestyle—with both parties working cooperatively, with our patients' understanding and involvement in this process.

～ Frequently Asked Questions

1. *What are the primary side effects of hormonal therapy that concern women?*

   The precise side effects depend on the specific drug. More generally, hormonal therapy tends to produce menopausal symptoms such as hot flashes, vaginal dryness, lower libido, night sweats, sexual dysfunction, and mood swings. These symptoms can be sufficiently severe to truly diminish a woman's quality of life. It is important for the health care provider to provide medications or other resources that can help reduce these side effects.

2. *What is the key issue to emphasize to patients who are taking hormonal therapy?*

   Providers must reinforce the importance of taking the medication as prescribed. Hormonal therapy drugs are taken for long periods and, therefore, are vulnerable to the same issues that arise with other medications prescribed for chronic diseases. In particular, noncompliance is an ongoing problem. The patient should be educated so that she understands the benefit she is receiving by taking the medication—namely, the reduction in her risk of recurrence of breast cancer; this message cannot be underemphasized.

3. *What can be done about the side effect of potential bone loss caused by AIs? Is a woman's risk of osteoporosis (e.g., because of family history or previous bone density studies confirming osteopenia) reason to not prescribe or discontinue an AI?*

It is increasingly common practice to prescribe a bisphosphonate for the patient to take with an AI, with the goal of preventing AI-related osteoporosis. Family history of osteoporosis or personal history of osteopenia has not been found to be a contraindication to taking AI as the hormonal therapy of choice.

4. *Which issues related to birth control should be discussed with a patient who is taking hormonal therapy?*

Even if her menstrual periods stop as a result of taking hormonal therapy (such as tamoxifen), the patient cannot assume that she is not ovulating. Therefore, birth control should be practiced by all sexually active, premenopausal women who are taking hormonal therapy. For women who were perimenopausal at the time they began their hormonal therapy, appropriate blood tests should be done to definitively determine their menopausal status before declaring that these patients are postmenopausal. Hormonal therapy carries a risk of birth defects if women become pregnant while taking one of these drugs, so the importance of practicing contraception should be emphasized.

REFERENCES

1. Miller NH. Compliance with treatment regimens in chronic asymptomatic diseases. Am J Med 1997;102(2A):43–49.
2. World Health Organization. *Adherence to long-term therapies: Evidence for action.* Geneva, Switzerland: WHO Publications, 2003:211.
3. Osterberg L, Blaschke T. Adherence to medication. NEJM 2005;353: 487–497.
4. http://www.cancer.gov/cancertopics/factsheet/Therapy/tamoxifen

5. Goss PE, Ingle JN, Martino S, et al. Efficacy of letrozole extended therapy according to estrogen receptor and progesterone receptor status of the primary tumor: National Cancer Institute of Canada Clinical Trials Group MA.17. J Clin Oncol 2007;25(15):2006–2011.

6. Buzdar AV, Baum M, Cuzick J. Letrozole or tamoxifen in early breast cancer. N Engl J Med 2006;354(14):1528–1530; author reply 1528–1530.

7. Wardley AM. Emerging data on optimal adjuvant endocrine therapy: Breast International Group Trial 1-98/MA.17. Clin Breast Cancer 2006; 6(suppl 2):S45–S50.

8. Loprinzi C, Stearns V, Barton D. Centrally active nonhormonal hot flash therapies. Am J Med 2005;118(12B): 118S–123S.

9. Kendall A, Dowestt M, Folkerd E, Smith I. Caution: Vaginal estradiol appears to be contraindicated in postmenopausal women on adjuvant araomatase inhibitors. Annals Oncol 2006;17(4):584–587.

10. Bender BG, Bender SE. Patient-identified barriers to treatment adherence: Responses to interviews, focus groups, and questionnaires. Immunol Allergy Clin North Am 2005;25:107–130.

11. Wirk B. The role of ovarian ablation in the management of breast cancer. Breast J 2005;11(6):416–424.

12. Joant W, Pritchard KI, Sainsbury R, Klijn JG. Trends in endocrine therapy and chemotherapy for early-stage breast cancer: A focus on the postmenopausal patient. J Cancer Res Clin Oncol 2006;132(5):275–286.

13. Goldstein LJ. Controversies in adjuvant endocrine treatment of premenopausal women. Clin Breast Cancer 2006;6(suppl 2):S36–S40.

Algorithm for Adjuvant Trastuzumab Therapy

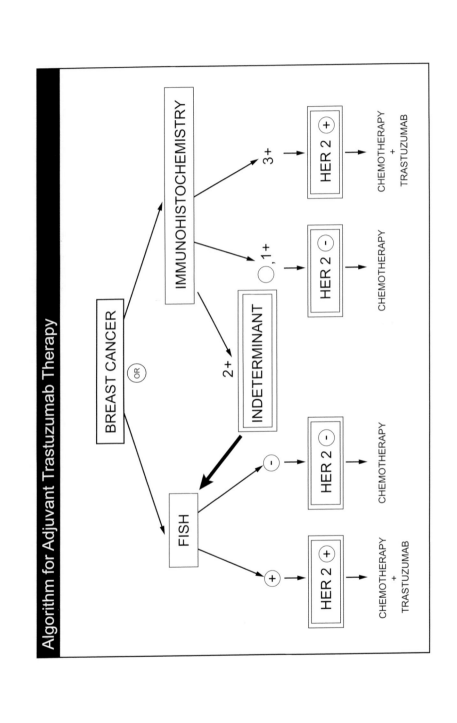

chapter

10

Monoclonal Antibody Therapy

Leisha A. Emens, MD, PhD

What you need to know:

Trastuzumab works in three ways: It can bind with the positive cell and block its cell division; it can attach to the HER2/neu-positive cell and signal the immune system to work, or it can work with chemotherapy (paclitaxel) to destroy the cancer cell.

Women with node-positive disease whose pathology confirms the tumor is HER2/neu-positive (+ + +) are oftentimes advised to consider trastuzumab therapy. This agent is given for a longer period than chemotherapy was; usually the treatments occur weekly for one year.

Approximately 5% of women taking trastuzumab will develop cardiac dysfunction, defined as overt congestive heart failure (CHF), cardiomyopathy, or a 10% or greater decrease from their baseline left ventricular ejection fraction (LVEF). Multiple-gated acquisition (MUGA) tests are done every 3 months during treatment, and an additional scan is performed upon completion of treatment.

It is not necessary for you to continue to do MUGA scans after your patient's treatment is completed and it has been determined that her MUGA results are satisfactory.

Targeted therapies for metastatic disease are also available.

*Dr. Emens has received honoraria for her participation in Breast Cancer Advisory Boards sponsored by Genentech Incorporated, the manufacturer of trastuzumab and bevacizumab. In addition, she receives research funding from Genentech.

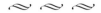

What your patient needs to know:

Approximately 26% of all women who are diagnosed with breast cancer will have HER2/neu-positive cancer cells and be candidates for targeted therapy.

Many women worry about the cardiac toxicity risk associated with such therapy. This risk is relatively small, and women are monitored throughout their treatment for these potential complications. In most cases, if cardiac toxicity occurs, it is reversible.

INTRODUCTION

Therapeutic monoclonal antibodies for cancer are targeted drugs that are highly specific for discrete determinants of a biologically relevant molecule associated with tumor growth and progression. Currently, two monoclonal antibodies—trastuzumab and bevacizumab—are commonly used for the treatment of breast cancer, and more are under active development. Trastuzumab and bevacizumab have unique side effects that fall under the purview of general internal medicine, so it is important for you to know about monoclonal antibody therapy for breast cancer so that you can effectively manage the patients in your practice who are receiving these agents. This chapter summarizes the indications and current data guiding the use of trastuzumab and bevacizumab to treat breast cancer, and reviews the toxicities associated with their use.

WHAT IS A THERAPEUTIC MONOCLONAL ANTIBODY?

Therapeutic monoclonal antibodies are genetically engineered antibody molecules that can be administered either to directly kill cancer cells or to stimulate the immune system so that it kills cancer cells. They are derived from the antibody molecules that are normally made by the immune system to fight infections. These proteins are normally made and secreted by B lymphocytes in response to stimulation by foreign antigens (protein, carbohydrate, lipid, or nucleic acid fragments) that are associated with disease. Antigens are substances that cause the immune system to mount a specific immune response.

The human body's immune response typically includes two components: a cellular component mediated by T lymphocytes and a humoral component mediated by B lymphocytes. The humoral component results from the secretion of antibodies by B lymphocytes. These antibodies are typically specific for multiple antigens associated with the particular infectious threat (bacteria or viruses) or disease process (autoimmunity or cancer). The humoral component is composed of multiple antibodies, each of which recognizes only one part of a specific antigen, but that collectively recognize both multiple, discrete tags within a given antigen *and* multiple antigens associated with the disease process. The diversity of the immune response is reflected in this *polyclonal* antigen specificity.

A *monoclonal* antibody is an antibody that is specific for a *single determinant* (epitope) of a given antigenic molecule. Therapeutic monoclonal antibodies are manufactured in large quantities in the laboratory rather than being made by the patient's own immune system. These molecules are produced by fusing a myeloma cell (a type of bone marrow cancer involving antibody-producing plasma cells) from a mouse with a mouse B lymphocyte that makes a specific antibody. The hybrid cell that results from this fusion is called a hybridoma. The fusion of a B lymphocyte that recognizes a specific determinant of an antigen with a myeloma cell that does not undergo senescence and death creates a permanent antibody production system, or antibody factory, that ensures a continual source of antibody specific for an epitope on a specific protein.

The potential drawback to this therapeutic strategy is that the monoclonal antibody produced in this way is a mouse protein, and hence will be recognized as foreign by the immune system of cancer patients who receive monoclonal antibodies as cancer therapy. To get around this complication, many monoclonal antibodies are genetically modified to eliminate as much mouse sequence as possible, thereby minimizing the possibility of a human anti-mouse (HAMA) immune response; the HAMA response can decrease the efficacy of monoclonal antibody therapy. Accordingly, chimeric monoclonal antibodies typically contain approximately 30% mouse sequences and 70% human sequences. In contrast, humanized monoclonal antibodies contain more than 90% human sequences and are highly unlikely to elicit a HAMA response. Trastuzumab and bevacizumab are both humanized monoclonal antibodies.

Two types of monoclonal antibodies are used in the treatment of cancer: naked monoclonal antibodies and conjugated monoclonal antibodies. Naked monoclonal antibodies can work in several ways. First, this type of antibody can attach to determinants on the cancer cell and mark it for destruction by the patient's immune system. Second, it can bind to factors secreted by tumor cells or other components of the tumor microenvironment, thereby neutralizing the influence of soluble factors that might otherwise promote tumor growth and progression. Third, it can attach to determinants on the cancer cell and block signaling pathways that might promote tumor cell growth and metastasis. Both trastuzumab and bevacizumab are naked monoclonal antibodies.

In a conjugated monoclonal antibody, the monoclonal antibody molecule is modified to contain a drug, toxin, or radioactive molecule. In this case, the monoclonal antibody acts as a delivery vehicle to direct the effects of the drug, toxin, or radioactive molecule to the cancer cell. In other words, it serves as a homing mechanism, searching out tumor cells for delivery of the therapeutic molecule directly to the site of disease. This approach has the potential both to maximize the therapeutic effect of the monoclonal antibody conjugate and to minimize the side effects of therapy with the conjugate drug. To date, no conjugated monoclonal antibody has been approved by the U.S. Food and Drug Administration (FDA) for the treatment of breast cancer.

MONOCLONAL ANTIBODY THERAPY: THE IMPORTANCE OF SPECIFICITY

The specificity of the monoclonal antibody used for cancer therapy is a critical determinant of its therapeutic success. This specificity depends in part on whether the monoclonal antibody is intended for therapeutic use in naked form or conjugated to specific drugs as discussed earlier.

For monoclonal antibodies that are developed specifically as delivery vehicles for drugs that can be conjugated to them, the specificity requirements are less stringent. In this case, the epitope specificity must track closely with the phenotype of the tumor cell to minimize the side effects of therapy and maximize its efficacy.

In contrast, for therapeutic monoclonal antibodies that are used in naked form, without modification, to deliver a therapeutic moiety, the antigenic specificity should reflect a target unique to a pathway that is critical and absolutely essential for tumor growth and progression. In this case, the antibody must be specific for not only the physical phenotype of the tumor, but also its underlying biology. For breast cancer, two naked monoclonal antibodies are in common use that target essential features of breast cancer biology. Trastuzumab recognizes the oncoprotein HER-2/neu, and bevacizumab binds to and neutralizes the pro-angiogenic molecule called vascular endothelial growth factor (VEGF).

BREAST CANCER SUBTYPES AND THERAPY

Breast cancer has been widely recognized as a heterogeneous disease for many years. Many mammary tumors are dependent on estrogen, progesterone, or both, for their growth and progression; these tumors typically express either the estrogen receptor alpha (ERα), the progesterone receptor (PR), or both. These hormone-receptor-positive tumors can be further divided into those that have a favorable or unfavorable prognosis using new assays of gene expression. A third class of breast cancers was defined when the proto-oncogene human epidermal growth factor receptor 2 (HER2/neu) was found to be overexpressed in 20% to 25% of breast cancers. Breast tumors that overexpress HER2/neu are typically more aggressive and are associated with a shorter survival.

These phenotypic and biological differences have major implications for therapeutic decision making. For example, expression of ERα and/or PR is an established predictor of response to endocrine therapy with tamoxifen, aromatase inhibitors (anastrozole, letrozole, and exemestane), and fulvestrant. Overexpression of HER2/neu is an established predictor of response to the therapeutic monoclonal antibody trastuzumab, which is specific for the HER2/neu protein dimer expressed on the cell surface.

TRASTUZUMAB: A HUMANIZED THERAPEUTIC MONOCLONAL ANTIBODY SPECIFIC FOR HER2/NEU

Trastuzumab (Herceptin) is a recombinant, humanized monoclonal antibody specific for the extracellular domain of HER2/neu that is exposed on the surface of a subset of breast cancer cells. This antibody is believed to induce its therapeutic effect by inhibiting cell proliferation, inducing cell death, promoting damage to cellular DNA, decreasing the production of new blood vessels within the tumor site, and recruiting the patient's own immune system to lyse tumor cells.

Trastuzumab was first approved by the FDA in 1988 for the treatment of patients with metastatic breast cancer who had been previously treated with one or two chemotherapy regimens. This monoclonal antibody was subsequently approved for use in combination with the chemotherapy agent paclitaxel (Taxol) as first-line therapy for patients with newly diagnosed metastatic breast cancer. Notably, the overall response rate for trastuzumab used as a single agent was 15% when the drug was given as salvage monotherapy, but increased to 26% when it was given as first-line monotherapy; median survival rates were 13 months and 25.8 months, respectively. When trastuzumab was given in combination with paclitaxel, the overall response rate increased to 41%, with a median survival of 22.1 months (compared to 18.4 months with paclitaxel alone).

The clinical trial studying the combination of trastuzumab and chemotherapy included arms in which patients received the doxorubicin (an anthracycline) and cyclophosphamide (AC) alone or with the antibody, or paclitaxel alone or with the antibody. Although the cardiac toxicity associated with the combination of anthracycline and trastuzumab is considered too high (as discussed later in this chapter), this trial is one of the few to demonstrate a survival benefit for any therapy in metastatic disease. It showed that the addition of trastuzumab to chemotherapy resulted in a statistically significant increase in the median survival from 20.3 months to 25.1 months.

Based on these data, trastuzumab is now widely used either alone or in combination with a variety of chemotherapy agents for the treatment of metastatic HER2/neu-overexpressing breast cancer. Current data suggest that the earlier trastuzumab is used to treat metastatic disease, the better the patient outcomes. Because it can interact synergistically with several types of drugs, trastuzumab is most frequently administered as the backbone of therapy in the metastatic setting. In this management strategy, the chemotherapy drug is changed at the time of disease progression, but the antibody is continued indefinitely. Patients with metastatic HER2/neu-overexpressing disease, therefore, may take trastuzumab for months to years.

More recently, four large clinical trials involving more than 12,000 patients demonstrated an unequivocal benefit to adding trastuzumab to the treatment of early, nonmetastatic HER2/neu-overexpressing breast cancers. Two of these studies [National Surgical Adjuvant Breast and Bowel Project (NSABP) B31 and Noah Central Cancer Treatment Group (NCCTG) N9831] examined the efficacy of four cycles of AC chemotherapy followed by paclitaxel weekly for 12 weeks or every 3 weeks for four cycles with concurrent weekly trastuzumab for 12 weeks, then trastuzumab monotherapy to complete 52 weeks of antibody therapy. The NCCTG N9831 study also included an arm that tested standard AC therapy followed by paclitaxel treatment, then trastuzumab for 52 weeks.

The third trial, called the Herceptin Adjuvant Breast Cancer Trial (HERA), allowed any type of neoadjuvant or adjuvant chemotherapy at the discretion of the treating oncologist, followed by observation, 52 weeks of trastuzumab, or 104 weeks of trastuzumab. For this study, the data on 2 years of trastuzumab therapy have not yet been reported.

The fourth trial was conducted by the Breast Cancer International Research Group (BCIRG 006). It studied four cycles of AC chemotherapy followed by four cycles of docetaxel (Taxotere) chemotherapy, a regimen that was compared to the same therapy with trastuzumab beginning at the time of docetaxel chemotherapy and continuing for 52 weeks, and to six cycles of docetaxel and carboplatinum with concurrent trastuzumab, followed by single-agent trastuzumab to complete 1 year of therapy.

Taken in the aggregate, these four trials showed that trastuzumab, given either concurrently with standard chemotherapy or subsequent to chemotherapy such that the total duration of antibody therapy was 1 year, reduced the risk of relapse by approximately 50%. The NSABP

B31, NCCTG N9831, and HERA studies demonstrated an overall survival benefit ranging from 24% to 33%; the BCIRG 006 data are too premature to reliably assess the overall survival benefit. Based on these data, the incorporation of 1 year of trastuzumab therapy into the adjuvant treatment of early-stage HER2/neu-overexpressing breast cancer is now considered the standard of care.

Data from the third arm of the HERA trial designed to examine the efficacy of 2 years of trastuzumab therapy will provide information about whether a second year of adjuvant trastuzumab therapy will provide an additional survival benefit. Furthermore, several small Phase II studies suggest that a short course of adjuvant trastuzumab, ranging from 9 to 24 weeks, may provide a survival advantage approximating that offered by the longer course of therapy. Further studies will be required to address these issues.

Predictors of Trastuzumab Response

The seminal trials showed that the level of HER2/neu expression is a predictor of response to trastuzumab therapy, with the highest level of protein expression being associated with the greatest clinical benefit. HER2/neu expression in breast tumors is most commonly characterized by immunohistochemistry (IHC) assays, which measure the extent of protein expression on the surface of the tumor cell. Alternatively, it can be characterized by fluorescence in situ hybridization (FISH), which measures the extent of gene amplification on the assumption that it might reflect HER2/neu protein overexpression.

Patients whose tumors express HER2/neu at levels scored as 3+ by IHC are considered candidates for trastuzumab therapy; those whose tumors express the protein at levels scored as 0 or 1+ by IHC are not. Breast cancers that express HER2/neu at intermediate levels by IHC, scored 2+, are considered indeterminate. These biopsies are sent for further analysis by FISH, which identifies an additional 24% of IHC 2+ tumors as belonging to the HER2/neu phenotype. All breast cancers with a level of HER2/neu gene amplification of twofold or greater as determined by FISH are considered HER2/neu-positive. Because FISH is not widely available, the common practice has been to first characterize HER2/neu expression by IHC, reserving FISH analysis for those tumors that score 2+ or are otherwise deemed indeterminate.

Safety of Trastuzumab Therapy

The pivotal trials of trastuzumab in both early-stage and metastatic breast cancer have demonstrated that this drug is generally well tolerated. The most common side effects are mild to moderate reactions to the first infusion of the drug. These reactions are characterized by fever, chills, and nausea, and are easily managed with acetaminophen and diphenhydramine. They typically do not recur with subsequent administration.

The most serious side effect associated with trastuzumab is cardiac dysfunction, defined as overt congestive heart failure (CHF), cardiomyopathy, or a 10% or greater decrease in the left ventricular ejection fraction (LVEF). This problem occurs in approximately 5% of patients who are treated with trastuzumab monotherapy, in approximately 14% of patients who receive trastuzumab in combination with paclitaxel, and in more than 25% of patients who receive trastuzumab concurrently with an anthracycline (the baseline rate with anthracycline therapy is about 8%). This high rate of cardiac toxicity with concomitant anthracycline and trastuzumab therapy led the FDA to approve trastuzumab in combination with paclitaxel, but not anthracyclines. Additional risk factors for trastuzumab-related cardiac toxicity include age older than 60 years, prior anthracycline therapy such that the cumulative dose exceeds 400 mg/m^2, preexisting cardiac disease, and prior chest wall radiation therapy.

The cardiac toxicity associated with trastuzumab is typically reversible. This characteristic distinguishes this side effect from the known cardiac toxicity associated with anthracycline therapy, which is typically irreversible. Anthracycline cardiac toxicity is associated with clear structural damage to the heart muscle, with myofibrillar disarray being seen on endomyocardial biopsy. In contrast, in patients who are treated with trastuzumab, the myocardium appears normal. The vast majority of patients who develop cardiac dysfunction while on trastuzumab have symptoms and signs of CHF, and improve with standard therapy for CHF. Most oncologists hold trastuzumab at the onset of cardiac dysfunction, and then cautiously reintroduce the drug once the patient has improved after taking heart failure therapy.

The adjuvant studies were designed to include careful monitoring for cardiac toxicity, and they specified clear rules for stopping trastuzumab therapy if the patient's LVEF dropped. In the NSABP B31 study, the cumulative incidence of cardiac events [New York Heart Association (NYHA) Class III or IV CHF and cardiac death] at 3 years was 0.8% (4 patients with CHF, no deaths) in the control arm, and 4.1% (31 patients with CHF, no deaths) in the trastuzumab arm. Corresponding data for the NCCTG N9831 study showed an incidence of cardiac events of 0.3% in the control group and 3.5% (20 patients with CHF, no deaths) in the concurrent trastuzumab arm. The rate in the sequential trastuzumab arm was 2.5% (16 patients with CHF, one cardiac arrest). In the HERA trial, the rate of symptomatic CHF (including NYHA Class III or IV events) was 0.06% in the control arm and 1.73% in the trastuzumab arm (1 year). One cardiac death occurred in the control arm. In the BCIRG 006 study, the rates of clinically significant cardiac events were 0.95% for the control arm, 1.33% for the carboplatinum-based trastuzumab arm, and 2.34% for the anthracycline-based trastuzumab arm. There were no significant differences between the rates of cardiac toxicity for the two trastuzumab arms.

The goal of treatment for patients with metastatic disease is disease control and palliation such that quality of life is maximized. In contrast, the goal of treatment for patients with early-stage breast cancer is cure. The established cardiac toxicity of trastuzumab makes it imperative to carefully select the appropriate patients who have early-stage breast cancer for this therapy by using IHC or FISH, and then to monitor them closely throughout the year of trastuzumab therapy. The current standard is to follow cardiac function serially with nuclear medicine multigated acquisition (MUGA) scans, documenting the LVEF at baseline and then every 3 months thereafter for the duration of therapy. Algorithms for managing the use of trastuzumab in the setting of asymptomatic or symptomatic declines in cardiac function have been published; CHF related to trastuzumab is managed according to the standard of care.

BEVACIZUMAB: A HUMANIZED THERAPEUTIC MONOCLONAL ANTIBODY SPECIFIC FOR VEGF

The growth, invasion, and metastasis of cancers depend on the formation of new blood vessels—a process called angiogenesis. VEGF is one of the key positive regulators of angiogenesis: It promotes endothelial cell division and migration, inhibits endothelial cell apoptosis, and supports the maintenance of the tumor-associated vascular network. Angiogenesis is known to play a critical role in the growth and progression of human breast cancers. The extent of the vascular network predicts the likelihood of tumor cell shedding at the time of surgery, the evolution of bone marrow micrometastases, overt disease recurrence, and patient overall survival. The central role of this vascular mediator in tumor growth and progression identifies it as a highly attractive target for therapy.

Bevacizumab is a humanized monoclonal antibody that recognizes all isoforms of VEGF-A. This antibody is believed to induce its therapeutic effects by binding to and inhibiting the action of VEGF, thereby reducing the extent and quality of tumor-associated neovascularization.

Bevacizumab was first tested as a single agent in patients with previously treated metastatic breast cancer. This patient population demonstrated a 9.3% objective response rate, with 17% of individuals being stable or responding at 22 weeks. Notably, 4 patients continued bevacizumab therapy without progression for more than 12 months. Given the relative safety and suggestion of efficacy, a randomized Phase III study then compared the efficacy of capecitabine (Xeloda) monotherapy and the combination of capecitabine and bevacizumab in 462 patients as second- or third-line therapy for metastatic disease. Although combination therapy significantly increased the response rates (from 9.1% to 19.8%), this increase did not translate into longer progression-free or overall survival.

Given the relative safety and the suggestion of efficacy as reflected by the improvement in response rate, a second Phase III clinical trial compared the efficacy of first-line therapy with paclitaxel and the combination of paclitaxel and bevacizumab in 715 patients with metastatic breast cancer. In this patient population, combination therapy resulted in an increase in the overall response rate from 13.8% to 29.9%; in those patients with bulky measurable disease, the objective response rate increased from 16% to 37.7%. An improvement was also seen in progression-free survival, which increased from 6.11 months to 11.4 months with the addition of bevacizumab to paclitaxel. These data are not sufficiently mature to give reliable information about overall survival, however, and the study remains in follow-up.

Based on these data, the combination of bevacizumab and paclitaxel is now considered a first-line therapy of metastatic disease for patients who are similar to those studied in this trial. This candidate population does not include patients with HER2/neu-positive disease, because trastuzumab is the antibody of choice for them. Randomized clinical trials evaluating bevacizumab as one component of adjuvant therapy for early-stage breast cancer that does not overexpress HER2/neu are now under way.

Predictors of Bevacizumab Response

The ability to select those patients who have the highest likelihood of responding to bevacizumab will be critical to minimize the risks of this therapy and maximize its benefits. This remains an area of active investigation. Two correlative markers that were examined in the study evaluating bevacizumab in combination with paclitaxel are serum levels of an endothelial cell-derived protein called vascular cell adhesion molecule 1 (VCAM-1) and urine levels of VEGF. To date, neither baseline levels of these markers nor changes in the markers with therapy have been found to correlate with response to bevacizumab.

Recently published results of a small, nonrandomized study evaluating bevacizumab administered in combination with weekly docetaxel as first- or second-line therapy for metastatic breast cancer identified E-selectin as a potential marker of response to bevacizumab-containing chemotherapy. Proving this relationship definitively will require investigation in larger, randomized studies.

Safety of Bevacizumab Therapy

Bevacizumab is generally very well tolerated. The primary side effects of this antibody include hypertension, proteinuria, thrombosis, and bleeding. These toxicities are generally mild to moderate in severity and are medically manageable.

The side effect of bevacizumab that is most likely to be treated in a general medicine practice is hypertension. In the clinical trial testing bevacizumab/capecitabine combination therapy, hypertension requiring treatment was observed more frequently in those patients who received bevacizumab, increasing from a baseline of 0.5% to 17.9%. In the study of the paclitaxel/bevacizumab combination therapy, the rate of hypertension requiring treatment increased from 0% to 13.5%. Hypertension is managed according to the standard of care both in patients who had preexisting hypertension prior to beginning bevacizumab therapy and in those patients who develop it de novo with drug therapy.

Clinically significant proteinuria and neuropathy (a side effect of paclitaxel) were more frequent in the antibody-treated patients in the study of paclitaxel/bevacizumab therapy, increasing from baselines of 0% and 14.2% to 2.5% and 20.2%, respectively. Algorithms for evaluating proteinuria and modifying bevacizumab therapy according to urine protein levels are under development but have not yet been standardized.

No differences were noted in the rates of thromboembolic or serious bleeding events in these studies. In clinical trials of bevacizumab as a treatment for other diseases, such as colorectal and lung cancer, more serious complications occurred (albeit uncommonly); they included wound healing complications, hemoptysis, gastrointestinal perforation, and arterial thrombosis. These types of events have not been observed in the breast cancer trials conducted to date.

LAPATINIB: A NEW TARGETED THERAPY FOR HER2/ NEU-POSITIVE METASTATIC BREAST CANCER

Lapatinib (Tykerb) is a new targeted anticancer treatment that received FDA approval in 2007. It can be used in combination with capecitabine for patients with metastatic breast cancer that is HER2/neu-positive. The combination treatment is indicated for women who have received prior therapy with other chemotherapies and targeted therapies, including an anthracycline, a taxane, and trastuzumab.

Lapatinib is not a monoclonal antibody. It is a small molecule that enters the cell to inhibit signaling mediated by the HER2/neu family of signaling molecules. Although it can inhibit signaling through both the HER2/neu molecule and the epidermal growth factor receptor (EGFR) molecule, current data suggest that this benefit is largely confined to breast cancers that overexpress HER2/neu. Lapatinib has activity in some patients who have HER2/neu-positive breast cancers that have been treated with trastuzumab and who are no longer achieving control of their disease with this drug.

The most common side effects associated with lapatinib include diarrhea, nausea, vomiting, rash, and hand-foot syndrome. Generally reversible decreases in heart function (which can lead to shortness of breath) have also been reported in a small percentage of patients.

Given that this drug prolongs the QT interval in some patients, electrocardigram and electrolyte monitoring may be indicated in certain patients.

CONCLUSION

Therapeutic monoclonal antibodies are changing the landscape of breast cancer treatment. Trastuzumab is already in wide use for the management of early-stage and metastatic HER2/neu-overexpressing breast cancer. Bevacizumab is increasingly used for the management of metastatic non-HER2/neu-overexpressing breast cancer, and it is likely to have a place in adjuvant therapy in the future. By virtue of their specificity, these drugs are highly effective, and each has a toxicity profile that is quite distinct from that of chemotherapy. The side effects associated with these monoclonal antibodies' use are typically mild and quite manageable. The toxicities that are more likely to require significant medical intervention are the cardiac dysfunction and CHF associated with trastuzumab, and the hypertension associated with bevacizumab.

Additional therapeutic monoclonal antibodies for the management of breast cancer are under active development, and their use is certain to further improve treatment options for patients with breast cancer.

~ Frequently Asked Questions

1. *My patient completed her breast cancer treatment several years ago and has done well. She is frequently on the Internet reading about new drugs that are available and is inquiring if she can now take trastuzumab, which was not available at the time of her diagnosis. What are patients usually told when they request treatment but we believe they are disease free?*

   This issue frequently comes up, because women want to feel more secure about their health and confident they have done everything possible to reduce their risk of recurrence. In general, women are not placed on targeted biologic therapy off protocol, and there are no data to support this practice. Remind your patient that she has responded well and that in the event that she were to have recurrence in the future, she can feel confident that new drug therapies such as targeted biologic therapies will be available to her.

2. *Patients are frightened about taking a medication that may be cardiotoxic. What information do you provide to patients regarding this risk?*

The doctor will make sure the patient has a strong heart to begin with by doing baseline tests (MUGA scan). In addition, the patient will be monitored throughout her treatment. Although cardiotoxicity is a serious event, its incidence is relatively low in patients who are taking therapeutic monoclonal antibodies, particularly when compared to the benefit these patients may gain.

3. *Limited therapeutic options are available for patients with brain metastases. Radiation is commonly given in such cases. What else is available?*

For women who are HER2/neu-positive, treatment with Tykerb may be a possibility, because this agent crosses the blood–brain barrier. This therapy is under active clinical investigation and is not currently approved for this indication.

FURTHER READING

Trastuzumab

Cobleigh M, Vogel C, Tripathy D, et al. Multinational study of the efficacy and safety of humanized anti-HER-2 monoclonal antibody in women who have HER-2-overexpressing metastatic breast cancer that has progressed after chemotherapy for metastatic disease. J Clin Oncol 1999;17: 2639–2648.

Ewer MS, Vooletich MT, Durand JB, et al. Reversibility of trastuzumab-related cardiotoxicity: New insights based on clinical course and response to medical treatment. J Clin Oncol 2005;23:7820–7826.

Keefe DL. Trastuzumab-associated cardiotoxicity. Cancer 2002;95:1592–1600.

Piccart-Gebhart MJ, Procter M, Leyland-Jones B, et al. Trastuzumab after adjuvant chemotherapy in HER-2-positive breast cancer. N Engl J Med 2005;353:1659–1672.

Romond EH, Perez EA, Bryant J, et al. Trastuzumab plus adjuvant chemotherapy for operable HER-2-positive breast cancer. N Engl J Med 2005;353:1673–1684.

Slamon D, Eiermann W, Robert N, et al. Phase III randomized trial comparing doxorubicin and cyclophosphamide followed by docetaxel (ACT) with doxorubicin and cyclophosphamide followed by docetaxel and trastuzumab with docetaxel, carboplatinum, and trastuzumab (TCH) in HER-2-positive early breast cancer patients: BCIRG 006 study. Presented at San Antonio Breast Cancer Symposium Annual Meeting, San Antonio, TX; December 8–11, 2005: Abstract 1.

Slamon DJ, Leyland-Jones B, Shak S, et al. Use of chemotherapy plus a monoclonal antibody against HER-2 for metastatic breast cancer that overexpresses HER-2. N Engl J Med 2001;344;783–792.

Tan-Chui E, Yothers G, Romond E, et al. Assessment of cardiac dysfunction in a randomized trial comparing doxorubicin and cyclophosphamide followed by paclitaxel, with or without trastuzumab as adjuvant therapy in node-positive, human epidermal growth factor receptor 2-overexpressing breast cancer: NSABP B-31. J Clin Oncol 2005;23:7811–7819.

Vogel CL, Cobleigh MA, Tripathy D, et al. Efficacy and safety of trastuzumab as a single agent in first-line treatment of HER-2-overexpressing metastatic breast cancer. J Clin Oncol 2002;20:719–726.

Bevacizumab

Cobleigh M, Langmuir VK, Sledge GW, et al. A Phase II dose-escalation trial of bevacizumab in previously treated metastatic breast cancer. Semin Oncol 2003;30:117–124.

Gordon MS, Cunningham D. Managing patients treated with bevacizumab combination therapy. Oncology 2005;69(suppl 3):25–33.

Miller KD, Chap LI, Holmes FA, et al. Randomized Phase III trial of capecitabine compared with bevacizumab plus capecitabine in patients with previously treated metastatic breast cancer. J Clin Oncol 2005; 23:792–799.

Miller KD, Wang W, Gralow J, et al. A randomized Phase III trial of paclitaxel versus paclitaxel plus bevacizumab as first-line therapy for locally recurrent or metastatic breast cancer: A trial coordinated by the Eastern Cooperative Oncology Group (E2100). Presented at the San Antonio Breast Cancer Symposium Annual Meeting, San Antonio, TX; December 8–11, 2005: Abstract 3.

Rosniak J, Sadowski L. Hypertension associated with bevacizumab. Clin J Oncol Nursing 2005;9:407–411.

Saif MW, Mehra R. Incidence and management of bevacizumab-related toxicities in colorectal cancer. Expert Opin Drug Safety 2006;5:553–566.

Lapatinib

Geyer CE, Forster J, Lindquist D, et al. Lapatinib plus capecitabine for HER-2 positive advanced breast cancer. N Engl J Med 2006 355:2733–2743.

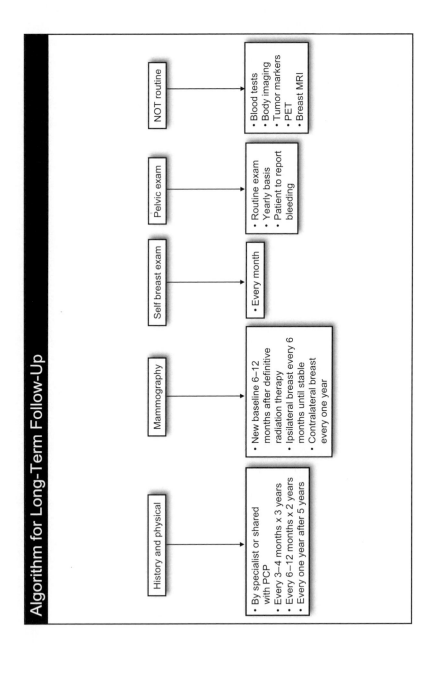

Algorithm for Long-Term Follow-Up

History and physical

- By specialist or shared with PCP
- Every 3–4 months x 3 years
- Every 6–12 months x 2 years
- Every one year after 5 years

Mammography

- New baseline 6–12 months after definitive radiation therapy
- Ipsilateral breast every 6 months until stable
- Contralateral breast every one year

Self breast exam

- Every month

Pelvic exam

- Routine exam
- Yearly basis
- Patient to report bleeding

NOT routine

- Blood tests
- Body imaging
- Tumor markers
- PET
- Breast MRI

11

Long-Term Follow-Up of Breast Cancer Survivors

Lillie D. Shockney, RN, BS, MAS
Charles Balch, MD

What you need to know:

Patients may show concern about not having scans and blood work done regularly after treatment is completed. The standard of care, however, is to rely on symptoms, and not to do scans and blood work once treatment is completed.

Patients' emotional needs may heighten during the first year after treatment is complete.

Chronic side effects may be the most worrisome issue that patients need your assistance with managing. These side effects may include peripheral neuropathy, cognitive dysfunction, and chronic joint pain.

What your patient needs to know:

The patient should make her doctor aware of any side effects that she is experiencing as a result of treatment so that the physician can better address the patient's medical needs.

Although it may seem unusual, routine scans and blood tests are no longer the standard of care for monitoring patients with breast cancer and evaluating them for recurrence of their disease. Instead, the patient should report any new symptoms that linger for longer than 2 weeks. At this point, any tests will be done if they are indicated.

The time required to recover from treatment—that is, the length of time before they feel well again—varies among patients. The patient needs to give herself that time, because breast cancer is a life-altering experience. She will be working to find her "new normal" going forward.

INTRODUCTION

During the surgical and adjuvant treatment period, patients with breast cancer are seen with relative frequency by their oncology team. Most teams will see the patient every few weeks, then progress to 6-month intervals, and eventually see her annually for some period. Once a patient reaches the point that her surgery, chemotherapy, and radiation therapy are completed, she is switched to a less intensive monitoring schedule, even if she is still taking hormonal therapy. In most cases, if the patient had her wish, she would continue to see her oncology team frequently just to ensure her peace of mind, even if no tests were done. There is a sense of relief when the patient hears them say that she *looks like* she is doing well.

As was mentioned in the forward to this book, women with early-stage breast cancer have the same health outcomes, whether they are followed long term by their family doctor or by their oncologist.[1] Given this finding, we may see increased pressure from insurance companies to have breast cancer survivors be seen for follow-up more often by their internists and less often by their cancer specialists.

Women who survive breast cancer—and the majority will—often find themselves without an organized system for maintaining their physical and emotional health. This is an issue that many cancer organizations now recognize and that the Institute of Medicine (IOM) announced in November 2005 that it wants to address. There needs to be a definitive plan for long-term follow-up for cancer patients in general. This chapter focuses specifically on breast cancer patients and your role in functioning as one of the key health care providers in their long-term survivorship care.

The IOM report confirmed that there is wide variation in how physicians track and care for cancer patients once they complete their primary and adjuvant treatment. "Awareness needs to be raised for both health care providers and the general public. It is common now for cancer patients to finish their primary treatment unaware of their heightened health risks. They are therefore ill prepared to manage their future health care needs," says Dr. Sheldon Greenfield, Chair of the IOM panel and Director of the Center for Health Policy Research at the University of California at Irvine.[2]

The IOM report recommended that cancer patients, upon graduating from receiving care from their oncology team, have a "survivorship care plan" that provides a road map of their history of diagnosis and treatment, plus long-term follow-up recommendations for primary care providers to follow. (It also recommended that both private health insurers and Medicare/Medicaid fund such plans.) For a woman who is completing breast cancer treatment, transitioning from oncology visits to routine follow-up appointments with her family physician and gynecologist is a significant milestone.

Figure 11.1 is an example of a form for recording a patient's breast cancer treatment plan. This treatment summary chart is also available on our website, and you are welcome to access and download the document for use in your own practice. To access a copy of this document for your personal office use, go to www.hopkinsbreastcenter.org, click on "library," and scroll down to the document entitled "Breast Cancer Treatment Plan Summary."* You can download this document and save it to your computer, if you like; otherwise, you can just print a blank copy as you need it.

It is recommended that you obtain copies of the patient's medical records directly from her oncology team, rather than relying solely on the patient being the source of this important medical information. Although some patients are excellent historians and provide accurate information about their treatment history, others (as you undoubtedly know) are not.

The breast cancer treatment plan summary is a document that can "grow" with the patient, particularly if you continue to see her during her active treatment. If you are assuming her post-treatment care, then this tool serves as the starting point for understanding her breast cancer history, prognostic information, and treatment she has

---

*In the "Post Treatment Issues" section of our website, you will also find a document designed for patients entitled "Treatment's Done—Now What?" Feel free to review this document and provide your patients with a hard copy of it.

Breast Cancer Treatment Summary

Patient's name: _____   Hx# _____

DOB: _____

Date of diagnosis: _____   Type of breast cancer: _____

Type of Surgery: _____   Date performed: _____

Pathology: _____   Tumor diameter (invasive component): ___ Grade: 1 2 3

ER: _____ % positive   PR: _____% positive   Her2neu: +   ++   +++

Sentinel node status: neg   pos   Total axillary nodes resected: ____   Total pos: ____

Chemotherapy: Drug given _____ # of cycles   Period of time given _____
Drug given _____ # of cycles   Period of time given _____
Drug given _____ # of cycles   Period of time given _____
Drug given _____ # of cycles   Period of time given _____

Radiation: Yes No   **If yes:** external beam   partial breast   full breast   chest wall   axilla
Period of time given: _____

Targeted therapy: Drug given _____ # of cycles   Period of time given _____

Hormonal therapy: yes   no
Drug given _____   Start date _____   Stop date _____
Drug given _____   Start date _____   Stop date _____
Drug given _____   Start date _____   Stop date _____

Other drug therapies: _____
_____

Recurrence: local   distant   **Where?** _____   **When?** _____

Other pertinent information: _____
_____
_____
_____
_____

Name of breast surgeon: _____   **Contact #:** _____
Address: _____
                                _____

Name of medical oncologist: _____   **Contact #:** _____
Address: _____
                                _____

Name of radiation oncologist: _____   **Contact #:** _____
Address: _____
                                 _____

FIGURE 11.1

Breast Cancer Treatment Summary

Patient's name: _____Jane Doe_____ **Hx#** _12345_ **DOB:** _10/20/1964_

Date of diagnosis: _2/10/2006_ **Type of breast cancer:** _Invasive ductal + DCIS_

Type of Surgery: _Lumpectomy with sentinel node biopsy_ **Date performed:** _2/21/2006_

Pathology: _1.8 cm total_ **Tumor diameter (invasive component):** _1.3 cm_ Grade: 1 2 ③

ER: _90_ % positive **PR:** _80_ % positive **Her2neu:** ⊕　++　+++

Sentinel node status: ⓝⓔⓖ pos **Total axillary nodes resected:** _1_ **Total pos:** _0_

Chemotherapy: Drug given _____Adriamycin_____ _4_ # of cycles Period of time given _3/06 – 5/06_
　　　　　　　Drug given _____ # of cycles Period of time given _____
　　　　　　　Drug given _____ # of cycles Period of time given _____
　　　　　　　Drug given _____ # of cycles Period of time given _____

Radiation: Ⓨⓔⓢ No **If yes:** ⟨external beam⟩ partial breast ⟨full breast⟩ chest wall axilla
　　　　　　　Period of time given: _6/06 – 7/06_

Targeted therapy: Drug given _____none_____ # of cycles Period of time given _____

Hormonal therapy: ⟨yes⟩ no
　　　　Drug given _____Tamoxifen_____ Start date _8/06_ Stop date _____
　　　　Drug given _____ Start date _____ Stop date _____
　　　　Drug given _____ Start date _____ Stop date _____

Other drug therapies: _____

Recurrence: local distant **Where?** _____ **When?** _____

Other pertinent information: _____
_____
_____
_____
_____

Name of breast surgeon: Dr. Thomas Operation　　**Contact #:** _(444) 555-1100_
Address: 11 Surgical Road
　　　　　Anywhere, USA

Name of medical oncologist: Dr. Mark Medicine　　**Contact #:** _(444) 555-2200_
Address: 14 Chemo Street
　　　　　Anywhere, USA

Name of radiation oncologist: Dr. Stephen Zap　　**Contact #:** _(444) 555-3333_
Address: Exray Parkway
　　　　　Anywhere, USA

FIGURE 11.2

completed. Figure 11.2 shows a breast cancer treatment plan summary for one patient.

LONG-TERM NEEDS OF PATIENTS WITH BREAST CANCER

Your patient's biggest worry is recurrence of her breast cancer. The majority of women who are diagnosed and treated for breast cancer live a normal life span. Although the incidence of breast cancer has risen from year to year in the last 15 to 20 years, the mortality rate has decreased. Women who have had breast cancer are at risk of getting the disease again and usually are aware of this fact. Twenty-five percent of women previously diagnosed with breast cancer will face the prospect of hearing "You have breast cancer again."

It is important to note that women who do get breast cancer again in the ipsilateral breast or contralateral breast do not have a worse prognosis or higher mortality than those who do not develop local recurrence or a new primary tumor. The younger she is, however, the longer her life and thus the greater her potential to be among the 25% of patients who reexperience this disease. Statistically, there is a 0.5% to 1.0% risk per year of a new contralateral breast cancer in these patients. Ipsilateral breast cancer recurrence may have the same prognosis as a new primary tumor in patients who previously had breast-conserving surgery.

Another potential risk is development of swelling (lymphedema) of the arm or breast. This problem occurs in 5% to 20% of women, with the risk depending on the degree to which the lymph channel draining the arm or the breast was interrupted after more extensive (radical) removal of the lymph glands in the armpit; the risk is greater if there was also radiation therapy to the armpit. For more information, see the American Society of Clinical Oncology (ASCO) website for patients (www. plwc.org) or the National Lymphedema Network website (www.lymphnet.org).

TAKING CARE OF THE WHOLE PATIENT

Taking care of breast cancer survivors involves more than just providing breast health follow-up. Rather, it means addressing the needs of the whole patient—both physical and emotional.

The leading cause of death in women older than 50 years of age remains heart disease. Although a breast cancer survivor may not be concerned about heart disease, she should be—if only because having had breast cancer does not make her immune to cardiovascular conditions. In some cases, her risk may actually have increased because of the side effects of some drugs used for treatment of her breast cancer. While a woman is going through her breast cancer treatment, sometimes there are lapses or delays in her annual or semiannual general health assessment. Assessments so affected may include her annual physical examination and gynecological examination; even eye examinations can fall off the radar screen.

The breast cancer survivor also has an increased risk of developing other types of cancers. In particular, the risk of ovarian cancer is higher for women with a diagnosis of breast cancer. Patients with breast cancer may also be at increased risk of developing other types of cancers such as colon cancer (see Chapter 14). Women who are taking tamoxifen should have annual pelvic examinations and Pap smears. If they report abnormal vaginal bleeding/spotting or other pelvic symptoms that cannot be explained, they may need further evaluation with transvaginal ultrasound and/or endometrial biopsy to rule out uterine cancer, as this condition is a known complication for a small percentage of women taking this hormonal therapy.

In addition, women on tamoxifen have a risk of blood clots. Thus a patient reporting unilateral leg pain, chest pain, shortness of breath, or other symptoms should be evaluated for deep vein thrombosis (DVT) or blood clots. In some cases, liver function tests may change while taking this hormonal therapy as well. Patients also need symptom management for hot flashes and/or possible depression (see Chapter 9).

Premenopausal women who have had ovarian failure associated with adjuvant therapy (chemotherapy) and postmenopausal women who are being treated with aromatase inhibitors (AIs) are at increased risk of developing osteopenia or osteoporosis; these conditions are associated with an increased risk of bone fracture. Bone health monitoring and bone loss prevention, therefore, need to be included in the patient's long-term management. If hormonal therapy with an AI is considered in women who have experienced amenorrhea following treatment, baseline levels of estradiol and gonadotropin should be obtained before the AI therapy begins, and the physician should subsequently perform serial monitoring of these hormone levels. For women who had bilateral oophorectomies before starting AI therapy, these blood tests are not necessary.

It is also important to assess your patient for adherence to long-term hormonal therapy, as compliance has proven to be an issue for breast cancer patients. Because the side effects associated with such therapy may overwhelm these patients, they may decide to skip or alter their dosing schedules in an effort to obtain symptom relief. This is a time to help them with reducing these side effects as well as to reiterate the purpose of the endocrine therapy. The goal is to keep these patients on track over the long term with the intended treatment regimen.

Many patients with breast cancer report feeling depressed after treatment is completed. In some cases, the depression may be related to losing the oncology team the patient saw as her touchstone, or it may be caused by side effects of hormone suppression, body image changes, or other feelings of loss (e.g., hair loss, symptoms of sexual dysfunction). Inquiring about the patient's emotional health needs to be part of every routine examination; you should not leave it up to the patient to bring up these concerns.

As described in the ASCO website for patients (Healthy Living After Cancer; www.plwc.org), women recovering from breast cancer are encouraged to follow established guidelines for good health. After a cancer diagnosis, many survivors may want to make changes such as eating better, exercising more, and finding better ways to manage stress. Although practicing healthy habits is important for everyone, it is especially important for cancer survivors because they can be at an increased risk for other health problems—for example, obesity, heart problems, diabetes, or bone weakness (osteoporosis)—as a result of their cancer treatment.

Patients need to talk with their doctors to develop the plan that is best for their needs. Moderate physical activity can help them rebuild their strength and energy level. Physicians should be prepared to help their patients create a safe exercise plan based upon each patient's unique needs, physical abilities, and fitness level.

ASSESSING PATIENTS FOR DISTANT RECURRENCE

Monitoring practices for metastatic disease vary widely among oncologists. There is general agreement on the need for physical examination every 3 to 6 months during the first 5 years and annual examinations thereafter. However, there are mixed views regarding which routine tests are beneficial. Some doctors order complete blood counts (CBCs), blood chemistries, and even blood tumor markers such as CA 27.29, carcinoembryonic antigen (CEA), and CA 15-3. The problem with the blood markers is that they are not sufficiently sensitive or specific to warrant their routine use in all patients. The most common marker used for breast cancer patients has been CA 27.29, which measures the presence of an abnormal protein associated with some cancer cell production.

Women who have had lumpectomy surgery and/or who have a remaining healthy breast should continue to receive mammograms. A new baseline mammogram is needed on the treated breast within 4 to 8 weeks after radiation is completed. Post-therapy follow-up is optimally performed initially by members of the patient's treatment team and should include regular physical examinations and mammograms. For women who are undergoing breast-conserving therapy, the first follow-up mammogram should be performed approximately 6 months after the completion of her radiation therapy.

National Comprehensive Cancer Network (NCCN) guidelines do not support routine ultrasound to screen the breast in asymptomatic patients. The use of dedicated breast magnetic resonance imaging (MRI) may be considered for post-therapy surveillance and follow-up in women who are considered to be at high risk of bilateral disease, such as *BRCA* gene carriers; the incidence of bilateral breast cancer is higher in women who carry the *BRCA1* or *BRCA2* gene. There is no evidence of any benefit from performing other imaging studies, such as bone scans, computerized axial tomography (CAT) scans, chest x-rays, or positron emission tomography (PET) scans, on a routine monitoring basis.

Bone density tests should be performed in women who are taking an AI or having some form of ovarian suppression or ablation. Be sure that your patient understands that a bone density test is not a bone scan and is not being done to look for metastatic disease.

A point of frustration for patients is the issue of not doing scans and tests on a routine scheduled basis. Some women prefer to have x-rays of some type periodically, even though they have anxiety about hearing the results. Based on information gathered by ASCO and the NCCN, there does not appear to be a survival benefit to finding the disease on a scan before a patient reports new symptoms of possible metastatic disease. Conversely, the ability to control the disease within the breast is surely improved, regardless of survival outcome. Studies published in 1994 confirmed that there was no impact on survival by doing intensive monitoring versus routine monitoring of patients.[3] Despite these findings, some doctors still opt to perform scans and measure blood tumor markers, although these measures are usually reserved for their patients who are at high risk for relapse or second breast cancer (e.g., those with locally advanced disease) and are employed less often for women who have early-stage breast cancers.

PATIENTS REPORTING CHRONIC FATIGUE AND REDUCTION IN PHYSICAL ACTIVITY

As many as one third of women treated for breast cancer have reported symptoms of fatigue lasting as long as 10 years after their diagnosis. The incidence was higher in women with cardiovascular problems and depressive symptoms and in those who were treated with combined radiation and chemotherapy. Although it is recognized as a subjective symptom, fatigue can be so debilitating that it affects the patient's quality of life and performance of activities of daily living.

In one study, researchers found that, much like in the first 5-year interval after diagnosis, 34% of women reported fatigue symptoms 5 to 10 years after their initial diagnosis.[4] Approximately 21% complained of fatigue at both time intervals.

Another study demonstrated that women who survived breast cancer accounted for nearly half of all female cancer survivors.[5] Overall these women reported high levels of health, physical functioning, and emotional well-being. Their energy level and social functioning remained the same as they were at the 5-year post-diagnosis mark and the 9.5-year remeasurement phase. In the follow-up study period, women reported less frequent hot flashes, night sweats, vaginal discharge, and breast sensitivity than they had experienced before. When the authors of this study looked at the late effects of chemotherapy, tamoxifen, or a combination of both therapies on quality of life, they found a statistically significant decrease in physical functioning associated with adjuvant therapy, even many years after the treatment ended.[5]

RECOMMENDED TESTS FOR LONG-TERM FOLLOW-UP CARE

The following tests are recommended for survivors of breast cancer:

▷ Annual mammography (for women who have not had bilateral mastectomies)
▷ Other routine cancer screening as appropriate for age and risk factors—colon, cervix, uterus

▷ Regular clinic visits for history and physical examination

Years 1–3: every 3 to 4 months

Years 3–5: every 6 months

Subsequent follow-up annually

▷ Health care maintenance: bone and cardiovascular health
▷ No routine tests—rely on new development of symptoms to trigger tests to be done
▷ Clinical breast examination annually by a gynecologist or primary care provider (PCP)

The following tests are *not* currently recommended by ASCO for regular follow-up care because they have not been shown to lengthen the life of a person with breast cancer:

▷ CBC and liver and kidney function tests
▷ Chest x-ray
▷ Bone scan
▷ Liver ultrasound
▷ Computed tomography (CT) scan or CAT scan
▷ Fluorodeoxyglucose-positron emission tomography (FDG-PET) scan
▷ Breast MRI
▷ Breast cancer blood tumor markers, such as CA 15-3, CA 27.29, and CEA

∼ Frequently Asked Questions

1. *What were the findings from the ASCO Expert Panel regarding surveillance of breast cancer patients?*

   The evidence supported the contention that the cornerstone for appropriate breast cancer follow-up is a regular history, physical examination, and mammography. The patient's history and physical examination should be performed by a physician who is experienced in the surveillance of cancer patients. Examination frequency should be as follows: every 3 to 6 months for the first 3 years, every 6 to 12 months for years 4 and 5, and then annually thereafter. Patients who are at high risk for familial breast cancer should be referred to a genetic counselor for risk assessment. For women who have had breast-conserving surgery, a post-treatment mammogram should be performed 1 year after the initial mammogram and at least 6 months after completion of radiation therapy. Routine tests are not recommended in asymptomatic patients.[6]

2. *My patient prefers to have a breast MRI rather than an annual mammogram because her breast cancer originally was not seen on mammogram. Is this acceptable?*

No, the standard of practice for breast cancer detection remains mammography. If the radiologist following her breast imaging studies believes that an MRI would be beneficial as an additional study to rule out or more clearly define something seen or felt, then MRI is used. MRI is not intended as a substitute for mammography, including for women with dense breast tissue.

3. *My patient has requested that she have blood drawn to evaluate for tumor markers at least every 6 months. She tells me it will reduce her anxiety if she can see that her blood results are remaining in the normal range.*

Tumor marker evaluation is not part of the standard guidelines for long-term follow-up and may be elevated for reasons unrelated to cancer recurrence. Because of their imperfect sensitivity and specificity, tumor markers are not routinely used to monitor patients for cancer recurrence. Educating your patient about this may help reduce her desire to have these tests. The down side of such tests is that the results may come back elevated without a known cause, which can increase her anxiety without good reason.

4. *My patient was on Herceptin. Do I need to perform routine cardiac tests on her over the long term?*

No, such tests are performed only if the patient develops new symptoms that trigger a need to evaluate her cardiac status. The oncologist should have performed left ventricular ejection fraction (LVEF) evaluations during her treatment and upon completion of her therapy.

5. *I do not know my patient's treatment plan for her breast cancer, and I do not feel that she is a good historian for this information. How important is it to know these details?*

Pretty important. You always want to know your patient's medical history, and this treatment is a very significant component. It is important for you to include in her medical record information about chemotherapy drugs that may have affected the patient's heart and the results of her last cardiac tests. Even knowing the details of the stage of her disease and, therefore, her risk of recurrence is necessary for you to provide your patient with appropriate care. If you do not have this information, contact her breast surgeon, medical oncologist, and radiation oncologist. Ideally in the coming years, as the IOM has recommended, a specific summary of this information will be provided to both the patient and to you as her long-term cancer survivor doctor.

6. *Where can I find more information and stay updated on changes related to the guidelines for long-term follow-up of breast cancer patients?*

Go to www.asco.org or www.nccn.org for the latest information on this subject. The ASCO website, www.plwc.org, is a good source for patients.

REFERENCES

1. Greenfield E, et al. Randomized trial of long-term follow-up for early stage breast cancer: A comparison of family physicians versus specialists care. J Clin Oncol 2006;24(6):848–855.
2. Institute of Medicine. *From Cancer Patient to Cancer Survivor: Lost in Transition.* Patricia A. Ganz, Director of Cancer Control, University of California, member, IOM panel; Sheldon Greenfield, MD, Director, Center for Health Policy Research, University of California at Irvine, Chairman, IOM panel.
3. Roselli Del Turco M, Palli D, Cariddi A, et al. The efficacy of intense follow-up testing in breast cancer cases. Ann Oncol 1995; 6(suppl 2):37–39.
4. Rodgers A. Routine follow-up of breast cancer in primary care. BMJ 1997;314:1129–1130.
5. Ganz PA, Desmond KA, Leedham B, et al. Quality of life in long-term disease free survivors of breast cancer: A follow-up study. J Natl Cancer Inst 2002;94:39–49.
6. Khatcheressian JL, Wolff A, Smith T, et al., for the ASCO Breast Cancer Surveillance Expert Panel. *2006 Update of Breast Cancer Follow-Up and Management Guideline in Adjuvant Setting.*

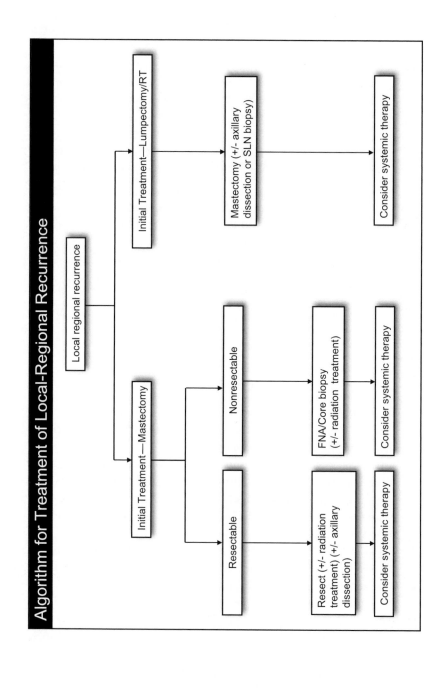

Algorithm for Treatment of Local-Regional Recurrence

Local regional recurrence

Initial Treatment—Lumpectomy/RT

Mastectomy (+/- axillary dissection or SLN biopsy)

Consider systemic therapy

Initial Treatment—Mastectomy

Resectable

Nonresectable

Resect (+/- radiation treatment) (+/- axillary dissection)

Consider systemic therapy

FNA/Core biopsy (+/- radiation treatment)

Consider systemic therapy

Algorithm for Treatment of Systemic Disease

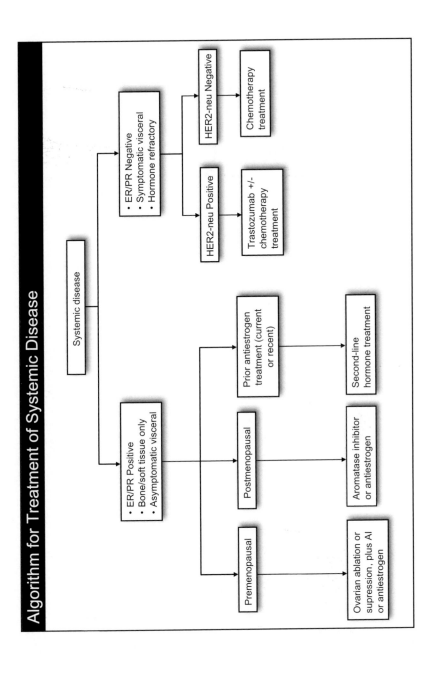

chapter

12

The Management of Recurrent and Metastatic Breast Cancer

Theodore N. Tsangaris, MD

What you need to know:

Local recurrence can be treated but should be considered a predictor of systemic disease and warrants consideration of systemic therapy.

What your patient needs to know:

Expensive screening tests and imaging are not appropriate for most women and do not improve survival from breast cancer.

Although a mammogram may have missed detecting the patient's breast cancer, mammograms are still the best screening tool for monitoring the breasts.

INTRODUCTION

Breast cancer is the most common malignancy in women. It is estimated that more than 210,000 cases of newly diagnosed breast cancer will occur in the United States in 2008. Cancer of the breast is the second leading cause of cancer death in women after lung cancer. More than 40,000 women in the United States die each year of the disease. Although the incidence of breast cancer continues to increase, mortality has been decreasing. In addition to the advances in screening and adjuvant therapy, this trend has been driven by a relatively recent (albeit modest) decrease in the rate of death from breast cancer. Nevertheless, however encouraging our treatment advances against the disease might be, women will still present with locally recurrent and metastatic disease.

Because of the greater use of breast-conserving surgery as the primary local therapy for breast cancer, clinicians can expect to see an increase in cases involving locally recurrent disease. Surgery offers an opportunity to decrease these ipsilateral breast tumor recurrences. However, systemic therapy in addition to local therapy is warranted for many of these individuals.

By contrast, metastatic disease is almost always not curable. The main goals of treatment of these patients are to control the disease, improve quality of life, and prolong life. Currently there are no absolute treatment approaches that work for all women. Generalized recommendations should be tailored to the patient and her individual circumstances. Clinical studies are defining the roles of endocrine therapy, chemotherapy, biologic therapy, and other novel approaches for treating metastatic disease.

SURVEILLANCE

In recent years, diagnostic testing for breast cancer patients has become more widely available. Traditionally, breast cancer follow-up has employed a conservative approach based on clinical examination and mammography. There is, however, marked variation in practice patterns, which can significantly affect the cost of delivering breast care. Equally important is the fact that excess or abuse of available diagnostic tools has never been shown to improve disease-free or overall survival rates.

Table 12.1 summarizes the current screening recommendations for breast cancer surveillance.

History and Physical Examination

All women should have a careful history and physical examination every 3 to 4 months for the first 3 years after primary therapy, then every 6 to 12 months for the next 2 years, and then annually thereafter.

TABLE 12.1 ～ Recommendations for Breast Cancer Surveillance

History and Physical Examination

By specialist or shared with PCP

Every 3 to 4 months for 3 years

Every 6 to 12 months for 2 years

Annually after 5 years

Mammography

New baseline: 6 to 12 months after definitive radiation therapy

Ipsilateral breast: every 6 months until stability is established, then annually

Contralateral breast: annually

Breast Self-Examination

Every month

Pelvic Examination

Routine yearly examination

Routine Blood Tests

No

Routine Imaging

No (includes computed tomography, positron-emission tomography, and magnetic resonance imaging)

Routine Tumor Markers

No

A word about examining the post-lumpectomy and radiated breast is warranted here. In general, the same principles of technique apply as when examining a breast that has not been treated for cancer. Examining the treated breast in the same systematic way the clinician has developed in his or her practice for examining the normal breast is very important. However, the radiated breast will feel different than the non-irradiated breast. Initially, post treatment, the skin will feel thicker and the breast parenchyma will be firmer. A residual mass or local distortion of the breast might be noted at the lumpectomy site.

Over time, the breast will attempt to return to its pre-lumpectomy and radiation state. Although they may never be completely normal, after treatment most breasts will look and feel very similar to the nontreated breast.

It is important to acknowledge the patient's concern that the treated breast might be difficult to monitor during the immediate post-treatment period. Reassurance, patience, and encouragement will be very important to the patient's acceptance of and comfort level with the post-treatment breast. Relatively frequent examinations provide both the patient and the clinician the opportunity to compare notes and impressions on the progress of the treated breast. These visits are beneficial to the clinician and patient in accepting and surveying the breast. In rare cases, the irradiated breast never progresses favorably cosmetically. These patients will be more challenging to monitor and will need special understanding.

Finally, although subtle changes in the treated breast are appropriate, discrete abnormalities that progress are never normal and always warrant further investigation.

Breast Self-Examination

All women should be instructed on how to perform monthly breast self-examination (BSE).

Mammography

Mammography should be initiated approximately 6 months after definitive radiation therapy for women treated with breast-conserving therapy. Subsequent mammograms should be obtained every 6 to 12 months while establishing stability. Annual mammograms should follow when stability is achieved.

Coordination of Care

Continuity of care for the patient with breast cancer is recommended and should be undertaken by a physician experienced in the surveillance of cancer patients and breast examination. Familiarity with and a level of comfort in the examination of the irradiated breast are very important. The primary care provider (PCP) may be the appropriate physician to assume follow-up care, provided that he or she meets the aforementioned requirements. The PCP should be expected to achieve results similar to those delivered by a breast specialist. A "shared-care" model of patient follow-up has been suggested and may be more appropriate, depending on the stage of disease and the requirements of long-term treatment such as adjuvant endocrine therapy.

Pelvic Examination

A regular annual gynecologic follow-up is recommended for all women. Patients on tamoxifen therapy should report any vaginal bleeding promptly given that they are at increased risk for developing endometrial cancer.

Breast Cancer Surveillance Testing: Not Recommended

The following tests are *not recommended* for routine breast cancer surveillance: complete blood count (CBC), blood chemistries, chest x-rays, bone scans, ultrasounds of the liver, computed tomography (CT) scans, positron-emission tomography (PET) scans, breast magnetic resonance imaging (MRI), and breast cancer blood tumor markers [CA 15-3, CA 27.29, and carcinoembryonic antigen (CEA)].

Management of High-Risk Women

Women at high risk for familial breast cancer should be referred for genetic counseling. These women include those with the following characteristics:

▷ Ashkenazi Jewish heritage
▷ Ovarian cancer at any age in patient or any first- or second-degree relatives
▷ Any first-degree relative with a history of breast cancer diagnosed before the age of 50 years
▷ Two or more first- or second-degree relatives diagnosed with breast cancer at any age
▷ Patient or relative with bilateral breast cancer
▷ History of breast cancer in a male relative

LOCAL–REGIONAL RECURRENCE

Ipsilateral Breast Tumor Recurrence

The use of breast-conserving therapy as the local treatment of choice for most early-stage breast cancers continues to increase. Studies suggest that patients who undergo such treatment have a 5% to 15% risk for ipsilateral breast tumor recurrence (IBTR). These recurrences are emotionally taxing to the patient and her health care providers, but definitely treatable. Most women who have had lumpectomy and radiation are best treated with completion mastectomy. Simple reexcision of the recurrence may be appropriate in selected patients and under special circumstances.

The significance of an IBTR appears to go beyond the immediate problem and anxiety of treating the local recurrence. Meta-analysis suggests that an IBTR is not the instigator of a patient's demise but rather a prognosticator of future systemic disease. For this reason, strong consideration should be given to providing any patient who experiences an IBTR with systemic therapy in addition to treating to the visible local disease.

Chest Wall Recurrence

There is no question that local recurrence of cancer in the chest wall, after initial mastectomy, carries a far more ominous significance than an in-breast tumor recurrence after breast-conserving therapy. The active search for metastatic disease is appropriate and unfortunately often fruitful. Systemic therapy is often used in this scenario. The presence of other metastatic sites, disease-free interval, prior treatment history, and performance score are all important factors when considering the multidisciplinary approach to these patients.

Nothing is more devastating to a patient than uncontrolled local chest wall disease. Therefore, when possible, a local resection with clear margins and radiation therapy should be utilized. If complete resection with clear margins is not possible, then obtaining tissue through fine-needle aspiration (FNA) or core biopsy is important in facilitating systemic therapy. Incisional or partial resections should be avoided, as retained tumor at the surgical site can make healing difficult, if not impossible.

Regional Nodal Recurrence

In the past, level I and II axillary dissection was performed with a lumpectomy, making resampling of the axilla for IBTR unnecessary and futile. However, the advent of the sentinel lymph node (SLN) biopsy as the standard of care has challenged this dogma. It may be appropriate to perform axillary dissection in IBTR for patients with a prior SLN biopsy. The more intriguing question may be whether it is appropriate to repeat SLN biopsy as a substitute for formal level I and II axillary dissection in these patients.

An increasing volume of experience reported in the literature has shown the success and accuracy of SLN biopsy for local recurrence of breast cancer after breast-conserving therapy. The absolute number of lymph nodes removed during the initial axillary sampling (which represents a surrogate marker for the extent of surgical manipulation and alteration of the lymph node basin) seems to be important when considering a repeat SLN biopsy. Studies suggest that reoperative SLN biopsy is more successful when fewer than 10 lymph nodes were removed in previous surgeries. Variation in the dye migration times and drainage pathways was also seen with increasing lymph node numbers. In addition to drainage to the ipsilateral axilla, lymphoscintigraphy revealed drainage to the internal mammary chain, interpectoral nodes, supraclavicular nodes, and contralateral axillary basin. For this reason, preoperative lymphoscintigraphy should be used before any approach to the axilla. However, as in cases of primary breast cancer, restraint should be implemented when sampling of the axilla will not influence subsequent systemic treatment or radiation therapy.

Internal mammary and supraclavicular lymph nodes are usually not addressed surgically. However, knowledge of their involvement could be important in determining the patient's prognosis and planning for systemic therapy and radiotherapy.

TREATMENT OF DISTANT METASTASES

The appearance of metastatic breast cancer is always devastating and almost never curable. Yet even in light of that disease dynamic, clear goals exist for managing patients with metastatic breast cancer:

▷ Cure the disease.
▷ Improve overall survival.
▷ Improve time to progression.
▷ Improve symptoms related to the disease.
▷ Improve quality of life.

In reality, the main goals in the treatment of metastatic disease are to control the disease, improve the quality of life, and prolong life.

As with adjuvant treatment, the clinician dealing with recurrent and metastatic disease must assess the patient for prognostic and predictive factors. Prognostic factors include an estimation of outcome independent of systemic treatment. This would be reflected in factors such as (1) tumor biology, (2) site of disease, (3) extent of disease, (4) time to recurrence, and (5) prior therapy. Predictive factors would reflect a relative resistance or sensitivity to a specific therapy such as estrogen receptor (ER) status or HER2/neu status. In addition, patient characteristics should be considered, including (1) age, (2) menopausal status, and (3) performance status (i.e., ability to perform daily activities of living). Finally, balancing toxicity and efficacy is always a concern for the patient and her health care team.

Clinical studies are constantly looking at the roles of endocrine therapy, chemotherapy, and biologic therapy in patients with metastatic breast cancer. Therapy options include the following:

▷ Endocrine therapies
▷ Chemotherapy
▷ Novel therapies
▷ Supportive therapy

These modalities will be discussed separately in further detail.

Endocrine Therapy

Approximately one third (67%) of patients with recurrent breast cancers will express estrogen receptors (ER) or progesterone receptors (PR). More than half of these women will benefit from interventions that modulate ER or reduce estrogen content. Therefore endocrine intervention should be considered as first-line therapy in women with newly diagnosed hormone-receptor-positive breast cancer.

A number of endocrine agents are currently available for use against metastatic breast cancer. They include the following classes of hormonal agents and other endocrine-based treatments:

▷ Selective estrogen receptor modulators (SERMS)
▷ Aromatase inhibitors (AIs)
▷ Estrogen receptor inhibitors
▷ Progesterone
▷ Ovarian ablation

Tamoxifen (a SERM) is effective in both premenopausal and post-menopausal women. Although tamoxifen has traditionally been the first-line treatment of choice for metastatic breast cancer, AIs' arrival on the scene has led them to challenge tamoxifen as the drug of choice in many situations. Several AIs have compared favorably with tamoxifen, even demonstrating some advantage compared with the latter drug. For instance, anastrozole, exemestane, and letrozole have all shown equivalence or superiority to tamoxifen in several studies in terms of both clinical response and time to progression. Of course, AIs are effective only in the absence of ovarian function. Therefore, in premenopausal women for whom tamoxifen is not appropriate, to reduce circulating estrogen the physician should prescribe ovarian suppression with or without an AI. Postmenopausal women should be placed on an AI.

Fulvestrant is a selective ER downregulator that acts as a pure antiestrogen. When administered intramuscularly on a monthly basis, it has been found to compare favorably to anastrozole in clinical trials; there are no significant differences in clinical response or time to progression for these two drugs. Fulvestrant has also been compared with tamoxifen as first-line therapy for metastatic breast cancer. Although the two drugs compared favorably with respect to time to progression and objective response, the clinical benefit was greater for tamoxifen.

The variations in the effectiveness of SERMs, AIs, and ER downregulators for particular patient groups merely emphasize the complexity of hormone therapy and the fact that there are several valid choices for therapy. In principle, the sequential use of hormone therapy is warranted. Studies are under way to examine the efficacy of combinations of agents such as anastrozol and fulvestrant relative to their efficacy as single-agent therapies.

Chemotherapy (Non-endocrine Therapy)

Nonhormonal therapy may be considered for the following indications:

▷ Hormone-negative breast cancer
▷ Rapidly progressing visceral metastasis regardless of hormonal status
▷ Hormone-positive disease that is refractory to sequential endocrine therapy
▷ Short disease-free interval following adjuvant treatment

Several factors need to be considered when choosing chemotherapy for patients with metastatic breast cancer. First, the relative benefits and toxicities of the various options for the individual patient must be considered. There are multiple options of treatment to consider, including combination versus single-agent chemotherapy, the role of dose-intense or dose-dense therapy, and biologically targeted therapy. Of course, while choosing an appropriate therapy, quality of life issues must be kept in perspective.

Several single-agent chemotherapy options have been effective as first- or second-line therapy. Of the popular classes of agents, taxanes and anthracyclines have been the most effective. With the increased use of these drugs in the adjuvant setting, the patient with newly diagnosed metastatic disease presents the clinician with a therapeutic dilemma. If the patient has been treated with an anthracycline or taxane in the previous 6 to 12 months, it might be preferable to start treatment with a different class of drugs. However, if a longer time has passed since use of these agents, then retreatment with an anthracycline or taxane might be considered. The availability of new forms of anthracyclines, such as epirubicin and the liposomal anthracyclines, has decreased concerns about cardiotoxicity and made retreatment with this class of drug for metastatic disease more feasible.

The question of sequential, single-agent therapy versus combination chemotherapy for the treatment of metastatic breast cancer remains an important issue. Combination therapy seems to improve response rates and time to progression. However, these benefits must be weighed against the greater toxicity associated with the combination therapy. It has also been difficult to prove improved overall survival rates for particular combinations. The following classes of drugs are used as both single and combination therapies:

▷ Alkylating agents
▷ Antimetabolites
▷ Vinca alkaloids
▷ Anthracyclines
▷ Taxanes
▷ Nucleoside analogs

Part of the difficulty in determining the benefits of single-agent versus combination therapy is the comparison of "apples to oranges." Many studies have compared one agent with a combination of different agents rather than comparing the same agents either in sequence or in combination. A recent Eastern Cooperative Oncology Group study (ECOG 1193) did use a crossover design, which allowed for the direct comparison of sequential, single-agent treatment and combination therapy. The objective response and time to progression were better with the combination therapy, but no statistically significant difference in overall survival was noted for single-agent versus combination therapy. Also encountered, however, were increases in grade 3 and 4 toxicities.

The correct choice of single-agent versus combination therapy might ultimately rest with the clinical needs of the specific patient. If a significant response is needed clinically, then combination therapy would be warranted. If the concern is minimizing toxicity without compromising survival or quality of life, then sequential therapy could be more appropriate.

Novel Therapies

Novel therapies for metastatic disease include trastuzumab (Herceptin), lapatinib (Tykerb), and bevacizumab.

Trastuzumab, a humanized antibody, targets and binds to the human epidermal growth factor receptor 2 (EGFR-2; also known as HER2/neu) in tumor cells. HER2/neu is a tyrosine kinase transmembrane growth factor receptor that is localized to chromosome 17q. Amplification or overexpression of this receptor is seen in as many as 30% of patients with breast cancer; it is correlated with a worse survival as compared with HER2/neu-negative tumors. HER2/neu-positive tumors have increased cell proliferation, demonstrate increased cell migration, and are resistant to apoptosis. By downregulating the HER2/neu receptor and reducing tumor cell proliferation, trastuzumab is effective as a single agent when used as first-line therapy against HER2/neu-positive cancers.

Data also suggest that there are synergies between trastuzamab and certain chemotherapeutic agents such as cisplatin, docetaxel, thiotepa, and etoposide. Cardiotoxicity again is a concern with combination therapy consisting of trastuzumab and anthracyclines, but less so with the trastuzumab/paclitaxel combination. Ongoing trials investigating the combination of traztuzamab and liposomal anthracyclines have shown encouraging reductions in toxicity while maintaining promising response rates. In addition, trials exploring the flexibility of dosing trastuzamab and the continuation of trastuzamab after first-line therapy are also under way.

Lapatinib binds to intracellular ATP-binding sites of HER2/neu and EGFR (ErbB-1), blocking downstream signaling. This dual blockade may be more effective than the single-target inhibition provided by agents such as trastuzumab.

In a Phase I trial of lapatinib and capecitabine, lapatinib was well tolerated and showed clinical activity. This drug has shown activity in trastuzumab-resistant breast cancer both in cell lines and in clinical trials.

Tumor growth is dependent on angiogenesis. Bevacizumab is a humanized monoclonal antibody directed against vascular endothelial growth factor (VEGF). It appears to have activity in patients with refractory metastatic breast cancer.

The emergence of new and novel treatments is an exciting and encouraging development for both patients and clinicians. Patients who would benefit from systemic therapy for metastatic breast cancer should be encouraged to participate in clinical trials when appropriate.

Bisphosphonates

Pamidronate and zoledronic acid are drugs that bind to the bone matrix and reduce the number of adverse events associated with bone metastasis. They also prolong the time to the first event. Patients with bone disease and pain experience a clinically relevant analgesic effect when they take these drugs. Given this fact, bisphosphonates should be given in addition to hormone therapy or chemotherapy for patients with bone metastasis, or to patients with a reasonable expected survival. These drugs should be administered in conjunction with calcium and vitamin D.

Bisphosphonates are associated with a range of toxicities. Renal toxicities have been observed, for example, so good renal function with close monitoring of creatinine clearance is important in patients who take these drugs. Osteonecrosis of the jaw has also been reported during long-term use of bisphosphonates.

Surgery

The role of the surgical oncologist or other surgical specialist in cases of distant metastatic disease is generally one of palliation. Although the decision to surgically intervene for palliation often has merit, the patient needs to understand that cure is rarely possible. The risks and benefits of any surgical intervention should be thoroughly explored by the patient and her health care team. Patients with isolated liver metastasis have traditionally been considered to have a poor prognosis, with median survival rates of less than 6 months. Several institutions have reported on use of the surgical approach in these situations. In studies with limited numbers of patients, morbidity and mortality are relatively low with modest gains in survival. Factors that favor a better outcome for these patients are hormone status of tumor, histologic grade, number of other metastatic organ sites, performance scores, and time to developing initial liver metastasis. Again, although some have advocated metastasectomy in selected cases of isolated lesions with reported improved survival rates, these scenarios are the exception and should be rigorously scrutinized on a case-by-case basis.

Radiation Therapy

As for surgery, the role of radiation therapy (RT) for metastatic disease is largely one of palliation. Radiation therapy may be preferable to surgery in such cases however, because of its ability to quickly achieve the desired effect on the disease and its avoidance of the morbidity associated with surgery. Brain metastases have increased in frequency, probably as a result of advances in palliative care. In patients with good performance scores and in the absence of multiple metastatic sites, intensified local treatment with systemic therapy appears to influence time to progression and overall survival.

The following are clinical situations for which surgery and/or radiation may provide significant palliation:

▷ Brain metastases
▷ Leptomeningeal disease
▷ Choroid metastases
▷ Pleural effusion
▷ Pericardial effusion
▷ Biliary obstruction
▷ Ureteral obstruction
▷ Impending pathologic fracture
▷ Pathologic fracture
▷ Cord compression
▷ Localized painful bone or soft-tissue disease
▷ Chest wall disease

In any case, the decision to perform surgery or administer radiation therapy for palliation should be undertaken only after careful consideration of the risks and benefits to the patient.

PALLIATIVE CARE

Statistics suggest that more than 85% of patients with advanced cancer will ultimately die of their disease. Although palliative care is now considered integral to the care of these patients, most patients are referred too late to get the full benefit of what is available. Unfortunately, many patients are never referred to palliative care at all. The World Health Organization (WHO) recommends that palliative care be initiated at the same time that therapy for disease is implemented.

The National Comprehensive Cancer Network (NCCN) Palliative Care Guidelines were developed to facilitate the integration of palliative care into oncology practice. Included in the guidelines are procedures for screening, assessment, intervention, reassessment, and after-death care. The needs of the family during this time and after death should also be addressed using these guidelines.

~ Frequently Asked Questions

1. *I feel discomfort in my treated breast. Is this normal?*

   Discomfort after lumpectomy and radiation is normal. The frequency and intensity of the discomfort should diminish significantly with time but may last a lifetime.

2. *Should I be getting a bone scan, CT scan, and blood test to see if my cancer is coming back?*

   Current recommendations are not to get expensive imaging and blood tests for routine screening. They have never been shown to improve survival.

3. *Do I have to undergo a mastectomy after a local (in-breast) recurrence of my breast cancer?*

   Most women with in-breast recurrences will require mastectomy. Special exceptions may be made for women with small recurrences, long disease-free intervals, and the presence or absence of comorbidities.

4. *Why do I need systemic therapy after mastectomy for a local recurrence?*

   A local recurrence is considered a predictor of systemic disease and warrants consideration of adjuvant therapy.

FURTHER READING

Carlson RW, et al. NCCN Clinical Practice Guidelines for breast cancer, v.1.2007. 2006. www.nccn.org.

Fisher B, Anderson S, Fisher ER, et al. Significance of ipsilateral breast tumor recurrence after lumpectomy. Lancet 1991;338(8763):327–331.

Gralow JR. Optimizing the treatment of metastatic breast cancer. Breast Cancer Res Treat 2005;89:s9–s15.

Khatcheressian JL, Wolff AC, Smith TJ, et al. American Society of Clinical Oncology 2006 update of the breast cancer follow-up and management guidelines in the adjuvant setting. J Clin Oncol 2006;24(31):5091–5097.

Levy MH, et al. NCCN Clinical Practice Guidelines for Palliative Care, v.1. 2006.

2006. www.nccn.org.

Luini A, Galimberti V, Gatti G, et al. The sentinel node biopsy after previous breast surgery: Preliminary results on 543 patients treated at the European Institute of Oncology. Breast Cancer Res Treat 2005;89(2):159–163.

Taback B, Nguyen P, Hansen N, et al. Sentinel lymph node biopsy for local recurrence of breast cancer after breast-conserving therapy. Ann Surg Oncol 2006;13(8):1099–1104.

Algorithm for Taking Care of Your Patient's Health

Emotionally

- Coping with fear of recurrence

- Differentiating between long-term side effects of therapy vs. symptoms of metasteses

- Support groups

- Stay informed about breast cancer therapy

- Psychotherapy if warranted

- Communicate with doctor about her concerns

- Participate in survivor retreats and events

Physically

- Exercise

- No smoking

- Avoid alcohol consumption

- Lymphedema prevention or management

- Nutritionally balanced diet

- Assessing risks for other types of cancers

- Stress management/yoga/relaxation

13

Psycho-oncology of Breast Cancer: Progressing into Survivorship

Lillie D. Shockney, RN, BS, MAS

What you need to know:

It is not unusual for women with breast cancer to have difficulty reengaging in their lives after their treatment has ended. This experience has been compared to the post-traumatic stress disorder experienced by some members of the military at war as well as individuals who are exposed to traumatic events.

Although most breast cancer survivors will have adjusted well after their first 2 years since diagnosis, 30% will not. These women may have issues with body image perception, fear of recurrence, sexual dysfunction, and stress disorders. In some cases you may need to refer your patient for psychotherapy to assist her with these issues.

More Breast Centers are offering survivor retreats for patients. These programs are designed to assist breast cancer survivors with lingering post-treatment issues.

Encouraging your patient to focus on the things she can control in her life, especially those that are health related, can greatly aid her in moving forward. These issues include weight management, smoking cessation, limiting alcohol consumption, and exercise. Encourage your patient to attend educational seminars to stay up-to-date on breast cancer and its treatment.

Make sure your patient is consistently getting her proper health assessments at the designated intervals, such as Pap smears, colonoscopy, physical examinations, vision checkups, blood work for monitoring her cholesterol levels, and other diagnostic assessments specific to her health issues.

Also investigate on the patient's behalf the availability of breast cancer support groups in her area and refer her when you feel it is appropriate.

What your patient needs to know:

Breast cancer is a life-altering experience. It is perfectly normal to feel anxiety when treatment has ended. Fear of recurrence is particularly common for most survivors.

The patient can regain control over her life (and health) by assessing her lifestyle habits and making changes where needed to improve her overall health and reduce her risk of breast cancer recurrence.

Patients should stay informed about the latest information regarding breast cancer and its treatment. They should rely on credible sources, however, and should not believe everything they find on the Internet.

Uncertainty can result in emotional distress. The patient should be educated by her medical oncologist so that she can distinguish between long-term side effects of treatment and new, persistent symptoms that might signal the need for additional evaluation.

The patient should be diligent in getting her routine checkups and health evaluation tests, such as Pap smears, colonoscopy, mammograms, and physical examinations.

Patients should stay active. It is one of the best ways for anyone to keep healthy.

The patient should speak with her oncology team about any programs the Breast Center may offer to help her transition back into her life. Many facilities now offer survivor retreats that can prove very helpful for patients.

Support groups can be helpful as well, but only if they are effectively moderated by a trained individual who knows how to facilitate such a group.

Some women may hesitate to celebrate their survivorship for fear it will jinx them. Your patient deserves the opportunity to celebrate. If she attends breast cancer walks and other events, she will undoubtedly encounter many other survivors there.

❧ ❧ ❧

THE PSYCHOSOCIAL TRANSITION AFTER BREAST CANCER

When a patient completes her breast cancer treatment, typically she feels more anxious than relieved (as confirmed by several studies). She is nervous about separating from her treatment team and lacks faith in her body because it has already betrayed her once. She also does not feel confident that she is, in fact, "a survivor"; there are even debates among patients and health care professionals about the point at which one can refer to herself as a survivor. If the patient is still taking hormonal therapy, she is technically still being "treated"—yet we do not think of her as a patient now in active treatment.

This is a period of psychosocial transition, defined as "major life experiences that require individuals to restructure their ways of looking at the world and their plans to live in it."[1] Some studies have compared this period to the post-traumatic stress disorder experienced by some military personnel who return from combat. Helping a patient achieve post-treatment personal growth is part of the physician's responsibility in assisting the patient to move on from treatment and reengage in life in emotionally and physically healthy ways. This type of psychological growth happens when individuals making positive changes recover from a traumatic life situation.[2]

The literature documents that the majority of breast cancer survivors have adjusted well after their first 2 years since diagnosis. However, there is a subset of survivors (approximately 30%) who report psychological distress, including depression and increased anxiety, 4 years after therapy ends. In addition, a large percentage of survivors report cancer-related problems long after treatment is completed, including concerns about body image perception, fear of recurrence, post-traumatic stress disorder, and sexual dysfunction.[3] These lingering concerns can result in a woman being unable to get on with her life as a breast cancer survivor. Each ache and pain is perceived as a possible return of the cancer. Studies have confirmed that this fear of recurrence centers on the possibility of death, future treatment, and threats to health, more than issues related to roles, femininity, sexuality, or body image.[4]

During her treatment, a patient was accustomed to seeing her oncology team frequently and being reassured that she was doing well and looked fine. At this stage, however, those visits are spaced many months apart and in some cases perhaps discontinued completely.

COPING STRATEGIES FOR BREAST CANCER SURVIVORS

This section describes some constructive ways to help your patient regain control over her life and move on from breast cancer.

The patient can assess her lifestyle habits and see if any are contributors to developing breast cancer. Smoking, alcohol consumption, weight gain, and inactivity can be considered contributors. By watching her weight, avoiding use of tobacco products (including secondary cigarette smoke), limiting alcohol consumption, and exercising regularly, your patient can feel more in control and see that she is taking charge of her health with steps that reduce the risk of breast cancer.[5, 6]

Staying informed about the latest research into breast cancer and its treatment is beneficial for many breast cancer survivors. This sounds simple, but your patient needs to be directed to obtain credible information, rather than simply accessing the Internet and wholeheartedly trusting whatever appears on her computer screen. There is as much misinformation on the Internet as there is valid information. Direct your patient to websites that provide accurate information and empower her so that she becomes an informed survivor. The website www.breastcancer.org is a useful resource, as is the Johns Hopkins site (www.hopkinsbreastcenter.org).

Some patients have difficulty returning to work and resuming their home routines, and they may need a bridge to help them for a while. There is nothing wrong with recommending that your patient consult a psychotherapist for help during this time. Breast cancer is a life-altering experience. Most marriages grow stronger when one partner has breast cancer, but some do not. Her family and coworkers may be weary after "holding down the fort" for months and, now that her treatment is done, they may expect the patient to be back to her old self and pick up all of her previous activities immediately. The patient is a different person, though—probably more in touch with her mortality. As a consequence, what she felt obligated to do before her breast cancer may seem trivial now.

Therapists and programs such as survivor retreats may help women set new life goals and figure out how to communicate with their family members about what they have experienced and how those experiences may have changed them. There is a tendency sometimes to seek a quick fix to such problems and get a prescription for antianxiety medicines. This is rarely the solution. It just numbs the patient and prevents her from dealing with the underlying cause, which needs to be discussed and dealt with openly.

Some patients experience difficulty differentiating between the long-term side effects of treatment (such as bone pain from hormonal therapy) and possible metastatic disease. Today scans are not routinely done as part of follow-up care, but rather new-onset, persistent symptoms trigger the need for diagnostic testing (see Chapter 11). The uncertainty can result in emotional distress for women who are trying to differentiate between symptoms from previous treatment and those that represent comorbid conditions, recurrence, or normal aging. Communicating with her health care providers may help reduce the patient's uncertainty in this regard and improve her emotional and cognitive well-being.[7]

Many breast cancer survivors worry about the risk of developing other cancers, such as ovarian or colon cancer. It is important to discuss with your patient those steps that can be taken to proactively monitor her health. Annual pelvic examinations, possibly periodic transvaginal ultrasounds in some cases, and colonoscopy in keeping with the standards of care recommended for other individuals will help her to feel more confident that she is doing well.

In some cases, a patient may limit her physical activity and not enjoy life as much as she could because of her fear of developing lymphedema. The advent of sentinel node biopsy has dramatically reduced the risk of lymphedema for patients who have been treated for breast cancer in the last few years. Those patients having axillary node dissections commonly are concerned about lymphedema, however, and there are mixed opinions in the literature about what may or may not trigger the development of this condition. One study supported the view that women treated for breast cancer with axillary node dissection, with or without adjuvant radiation therapy, could maintain their level of physical activity and occupational workload after treatment without an added risk of developing arm lymphedema. Having a higher body mass index (BMI) before and after the surgery appears to increase the risk of lymphedema, however.[8]

Some women experience great anxiety and guilt, fearing they may have passed this disease to their children. For women who may carry a breast cancer gene, this is a time to discuss and possibly refer them for genetic evaluation (see Chapter 14). If your patient does carry a breast cancer gene, encourage her to discuss with a genetics counselor ways to further assess her children's risk, if necessary. A breast cancer gene is no one's fault; it was not planned. This message sometimes needs to be reiterated to assuage a patient's feelings of guilt.

Anxiety about having "missed" the benefits of newer treatment options that were developed and became available after their treatment was completed is an issue for some patients. Women may read about new drugs and new treatments and feel deprived because these options were not available when they had treatment. Some will even attempt to find a doctor who would be willing to give them the treatment now, even if it has been several years since their breast cancer diagnosis and treatment. Providers need to emphasize that these treatments will be available if patients need them in the future as well as explain that there are women who were diagnosed in even earlier generations who also wish they had the treatments that these women received more recently. The good news is that there are new treatments being developed on an ongoing basis that will benefit the next generation.

Encourage your patients to participate in breast cancer events that celebrate survivorship and raise money for breast cancer research. Having survivors come together for a common cause is good for everyone. Seeing others who feel the way they do reassures survivors that they are not alone in their concerns. Raising money for research helps them to feel more positive about the outlook for the next generation—perhaps less treatment, and perhaps even prevention and cure.

Support groups have both good features and not-so-good features. Women who are going through active treatment can benefit from talking with others who are doing the same as well as women who have recently completed their treatment. They can feel camaraderie, a sense of belonging, and be reassured that the thoughts and fears that they are experiencing are normal. Women who attend support groups for many years, however, may not be doing themselves any favors. Most women find it difficult to strike a balance between wanting emotional support and wanting to be treated as normal. In one study, organized support groups were helpful to only 13% of those surveyed.[9] For some women, these groups may actually promote fear of recurrence. How effective the facilitator is in running the support group is critical to its success in helping women with their emotional well-being. If a woman is 10 years out from treatment and still feels a need to be in a support group and talk about her fears, then it may be a signal that she needs one-on-one psychotherapy.

Make your patients aware when an educational seminar is available in your area to update them on breast cancer diagnosis and treatment. This kind of event is something that many survivors enjoy attending, and they appreciate their doctors and nurses letting them know about these meetings. Such seminars help to reduce fear for most women and keep them informed about what is the latest news regarding diagnosis, treatment, and the future as it relates to preventing and finding a cure for breast cancer.

Finally, sending your patient information via mail about self-promoting good lifestyle habits is something that patients welcome, according to a study that focused on patients' readiness to pursue lifestyle changes to improve their health.[10]

⁓ Frequently Asked Questions

1. *What is the number one issue of concern for women after completion of their adjuvant therapy?*

   Most breast cancer survivors fear recurrence of the disease—both local recurrence and, even more so, distant recurrence that would place them in a stage IV situation. Women need a lot of reassurance regarding this issue and accurate statistics to put their risk of recurrence into perspective; otherwise, patients can end up being controlled by this disease even though they have beaten it.

2. *What are patients' other major concerns?*

   Some patients fear that they may have passed the risk of getting breast cancer on to their children (via a breast cancer gene). Women need to be educated about genetic risk and be evaluated for it as part of their initial assessment at the time of diagnosis. The majority of women diagnosed with breast cancer will not carry the *BRCA1* or *BRCA2* gene; in such cases, their disease did not have a genetic origin. Helping a patient understand what the risk is for her children based on genetic risk versus not being connected to hereditary causes is important. Both the patient and her children will rest easier with this understanding. (See Chapter 14 for more information about genetic risk.)

3. *What are constructive things women can do to reduce their risk of recurrence once they have been diagnosed and treated for breast cancer?*

Breast cancer survivors should watch their diet—a low-fat diet is recommended. Exercise regularly. No smoking. Limit alcohol intake. Do not take hormone replacement therapy (HRT).

4. *What are other ways to reduce anxiety about breast cancer for women who have had this disease or fear getting it?*

There is power in information. Keeping your patient informed of the latest research findings and progress related to breast cancer diagnosis, treatment, and prevention is helpful to her. Directing her to credible websites and newsletters about breast cancer is wise. Discourage your patient from seeking information from just any website, as some information found on the Internet is inaccurate and can produce more fear and misunderstanding.

REFERENCES

1. Parkes CM. Psycho-social transitions: A field for study. Social Sci Med 1998;5:101–115.
2. Tedeschi RG, Calhoun LG. The Post-traumatic Growth Inventory: Measuring the positive legacy of trauma. J Traum Stress 1996;9:455–471.
3. Kornblith AB, Ligibel J. Psychosocial and sexual functioning of survivors of breast cancer. Semin Oncol 2003;30(6):799–813.
4. Vickberg SM. The concerns about recurrence scales (CARS): A systematic measure of women's fears about the possibility of breast cancer recurrence. Ann Behav Med 2003;25(1):16–24.
5. Fentiman IS, Allen DS, Hamed H. Smoking and prognosis in women with breast cancer. Intl J Clin Pract 2005;59(9):999–1000.

6. Thomson CA, Flatt SW, Rock CL, et al. Increased fruit, vegetable and fiber intake and lower fat intake reported among women previously treated for invasive breast cancer. J Am Diet Assoc 2002;102(6):801–808.

7. Clayton MF, Mishel MH, Belyea M. Testing a model of symptoms, communication, uncertainty, and well-being in older breast cancer survivors. Res Nurs Health 2006;29(1):18–39.

8. Johansson K, Ohlsson K, Ingvar C, et al. Factors associated with the development of arm lymphedema following breast cancer treatment: A match pair case control study. Lymphology 2002;35(2);59–71.

9. Chantler M, Podbilewicz-Schuller Y, Mortimer J. Change in need for psychosocial support for women with early stage breast cancer. J Psychosoc Oncol 2005;23(2–3):65–77.

10. Demark-Wahnefried W, Peterson B, McBride C, et al. Current health behaviors and readiness to pursue life style changes among men and women diagnosed with early stage prostate and breast carcinomas. Cancer 2000;88(3):674–684.

Algorithm for Women at High Risk

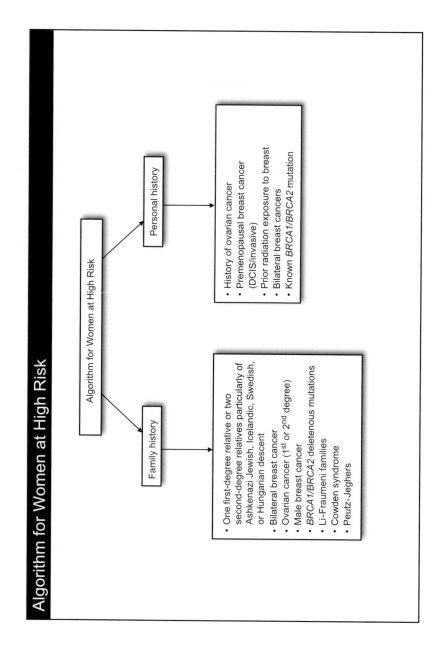

chapter

14

A Practical Approach to Assessing High-Risk Women

Kala Visvanathan MD, BS, FRACP, MHS

What you need to know:

If you are considering referring a patient for assessment of breast cancer risk factors (which may include genetic testing), screening, and risk-reduction options owing to family or personal history, plan to provide the following medical information so that the doctor and genetic counselor seeing her can accurately do the assessment requested:

▷ Family history of breast cancer in a first- or second-degree relative

▷ Detailed gynecologic and breast surgical history, as well as radiological history

▷ Medical history including risk factors—age at first menstrual period, age at menopause, age at birth of first child, history of atypical hyperplasia, history of breast biopsies, race, knowledge of prior genetic testing in her family, personal history of cancers

Although 20% to 30% of women may have a family history of breast cancer, only 5% to 10% have a hereditary predisposition toward this disease.

Women who carry deleterious mutations in the *BRCA1* or *BRCA2* genes are counseled about preventive steps to take to reduce their risk of developing cancer. Their risk during the lifetime is 36% to 85%; more detailed risk estimates are available based on age. Women are currently recommended to undergo prophylactic oophorectomy if they are past childbearing because of the limited specificity of current screening methods for ovarian cancer. In terms of breast cancer risk, options that are discussed with patients include increased screening [i.e., clinical breast examinations, mammograms, breast magnetic resonance imaging (MRI)], chemoprevention (tamoxifen), and prophylactic mastectomy. Data on the frequency and timing of MRI in such cases are currently being gathered. Based on existing data, however, it appears that prophylactic mastectomy can reduce the risk of breast cancer in high-risk women by 95%; prophylactic oophorectomy can reduce the risk by 80% to 90%.

Certain familial syndromes are associated with a higher risk of breast cancer, in addition to the deleterious mutations in the *BRCA1* and *BRCA2* genes. These conditions include Li-Fraumeni syndrome, Cowden syndrome, and Peutz-Jeghers syndrome.

There are specific clues that may be present in unaffected women, raising the possibility of them carrying a breast cancer gene. Table 14.1 lists these characteristics.

TABLE 14.1   ∽   **Risk Factors for Breast Cancer**

The following findings are important clues in women who are as yet unaffected by breast cancer, but who may have an inherited predisposition to breast cancer based on the family history of first- and second-degree relatives on either the maternal or paternal side, or both:

More than one relative with early-onset breast cancer (younger than 50 years old)

Bilateral breast cancer

Male breast cancer

Ovarian cancer at any age

Breast and ovarian cancer in the same individual; bilateral breast cancer

One relative with breast and/or ovarian cancer if the individual has any of the following ethnic backgrounds in whom founder mutations have been identified: Ashkenazi Jewish, Icelandic, Swedish, Hungarian

Family member with a known genetic mutation in a breast cancer susceptibility gene

History of multiple family members with pancreatic cancer, melanoma, prostate cancer, or gastric cancer

Cancer clusters of the following (not every cancer may be seen in the pedigree):

▷ Early-onset breast cancer, osteosarcoma, leukemia, brain tumors, adrenocortical malignancies, endometrial cancer (Li-Fraumeni syndrome)

▷ Early-onset breast cancer, nonmedullary thyroid cancer/ benign thyroid follicular adenoma or multinodular goiter; multiple hamartomatous lesions in skin (often at age 20 years), intestine, oral mucosa, or breast; prior history of benign breast disease (Cowden syndrome)

▷ Early-onset breast cancer; hamartomous polyps in gastrointestinal tract; melanin deposits in buccal mucosa, lips, fingers, and toes (Peutz-Jeghers syndrome)

What your patient needs to know:

Your patient does not have control over her heredity and genetic make-up but she does have control over how she addresses her high-risk status.

Many women assume if they have a relative anywhere in their family tree with breast cancer, they are destined to get breast cancer. In fact, most women with a family history will not get this disease. Those at higher risk often have a family history that includes a first-degree relative or at least two second-degree relatives who were diagnosed at a relatively young age with breast cancer.

Genetic counseling and testing is available for two specific tumor suppressor genes—*BRCA1* and *BRCA2*. Other, less penetrant genes are likely to be identified in the future as factors in breast cancer development. Thus, if a woman's family history fits a specific pattern or she has developed breast cancer at an early age or has a history of ovarian cancer, she should be referred to a high-risk breast clinic for consideration of genetic testing. Where possible, genetic testing is undertaken on the person who is affected by breast cancer; if her test for the mutation is positive, then other healthy family members may undergo testing.

Women need genetic counseling and discussion of their risk before they embark on genetic testing. Although the test itself is simply a blood test, the ramifications of the results of the test need careful discussion before those results become known. For example, if testing would not change the patient's current management or be helpful for family members, then she might decide to postpone the test.

Certain syndromes put some women at higher risk for hereditary breast cancer. Having hereditary breast cancer may increase the risk of other types of cancers, such as ovarian cancer.

～ ～ ～

INTRODUCTION

This chapter is intended as a review of current clinical approaches used to identify healthy women at high risk for breast cancer to assist physicians and other health providers in giving risk-appropriate screening and management recommendations. Knowledge of a woman's breast cancer risk can be used to guide both screening and risk-reduction strategies. Such information can also decrease anxiety, particularly in young women with risk factors such as family history, as their perceived risk of developing breast cancer is often much higher than their actual risk. The overall goal of breast cancer risk assessment is twofold: (1) to target high risk groups with more aggressive screening and risk-reduction strategies so as to increase their overall survival and (2) to minimize overtreatment and its associated complications in low-risk groups.

At any age a woman can be classified as being at general population risk, at increased risk, or at high risk for breast cancer. The following medical, surgical, and family history information is needed to determine which risk group a woman fits into:

▷ Family history of cancer in first- and second-degree relatives on both the maternal and paternal sides
▷ Detailed gynecological and breast surgical history
▷ Medical history, including known breast cancer risk factors such as age at menarche, parity, age at birth of first child, age at

menopause (if occurred), history of previous breast biopsies, history of atypical hyperplasia, and race (in particular, whether there is any Ashkenazi Jewish heritage)

▷ Knowledge of any prior genetic testing in the family

▷ Information on any personal history of cancer

In practice, patients often may not remember or be able to provide this information immediately if asked at a clinic visit, particularly family history. Therefore, requesting this information prior to the patient's appointment can be extremely helpful and efficient, and it can result in a more comprehensive and accurate assessment.

It is reasonable to perform a baseline risk assessment when a woman is between the ages of 18 and 20 years to determine whether she has a strong family history of breast cancer or possible hereditary syndrome that might affect her breast cancer risk. Early identification of these women with a hereditary predisposition toward breast cancer is important, as they need to be more closely monitored with intense surveillance throughout their lifetime and may benefit from genetic testing and targeted risk-reduction strategies in their twenties. A woman's breast cancer risk should be regularly reevaluated over her lifetime, because many of the known risk factors (including family history and age) will change over time and with the woman's experiences.

IDENTIFICATION OF WOMEN AT HIGH RISK
FOR BREAST CANCER

Family history of breast cancer is an important risk factor on its own. A woman with a first-degree relative with breast cancer has a two- to threefold increased risk of developing breast cancer as compared to women with no such family history. This risk increases to fourfold if there is more than one first-degree relative with breast cancer. Although 20% to 30% of women report having at least one relative with breast cancer, only 5% to 10% have what is known as a hereditary predisposition, which places them at high risk for breast cancer (Table 14.2). For women with any one of these rare inherited syndromes, the risk of developing breast cancer in their lifetime ranges from 22% to 85%. Age-specific estimates of this risk play an

TABLE 14.2 〜 Inherited Syndromes Associated with a High Risk of Early-Onset Breast Cancer

Familial Syndrome	Gene Involved	Other Associated Conditions
Breast/ovarian	BRCA1/BRCA2	Ovarian, pancreas, prostate, melanoma, and male breast cancers
Li-Fraumeni syndrome	p53	Bone or soft-tissue sarcoma, leukemia, brain tumors, and adrenocortical malignancies, childhood cancers, adenocarcinoma
Cowden syndrome	PTEN	Mucocutaneous lesions of the face and oral mucosa, cerebellar tumors, benign and malignant (nonmedullary) thyroid cancer, endometrial cancer, macrocephaly, mental retardation, multiple hamartomas of the gastrointestinal tract, uterine fibromas, benign breast lesions, lipomas
Peutz-Jeghers syndrome	STK11	Hamartomous polyps in gastrointestinal tract; freckles in buccal mucosa, lips, fingers, and toes; thyroid cancer; ovarian cancer including sex cord tumors

important role when discussing management options. These women are also at risk for other cancers and related benign conditions. The chance that they develop at least one type of cancer in their lifetime is close to 90%.

BRCA Genes

The majority of known hereditary breast cancers are due to deleterious mutations in the *BRCA1* and *BRCA2* genes. These tumor suppressor genes are involved in DNA repair. The *BRCA1* gene is located on chromosome 17, and the *BRCA2* gene is found on chromosome 13. An individual has two copies of each gene, one from each parent. Deleterious mutations in each gene are inherited in an autosomal dominant manner. Mutations in BRCA1 are thought to explain 90% of breast and ovarian cancers observed in families and 45% of multiple breast cancer cases.

In the general population, the prevalence of *BRCA* mutations is rare, occurring in 0.1% of women. Specific familial mutations in these genes are more common in certain populations, such as Ashkenazi Jewish women. The lifetime risk of breast cancer among women who are mutation carriers has been estimated to be between 36% and 85%, according to reported studies from different study populations. The lifetime risk of ovarian cancer is between 16% and 60% in the same population. Mutation carriers also have an increased risk of second breast cancers. Men with deleterious mutations in these two genes are also at increased risk for male breast cancer and prostate cancer, albeit to a lesser degree. Melanoma and pancreatic cancers in some families have also been linked to these mutations.

Genetic testing for mutations in these two genes is available. Screening guidelines have been developed for *BRCA* mutation carriers based on the opinions of expert groups. Young women in families in which there is a known mutation should be encouraged to perform breast self-examinations from the age 18 years onward; from age 25 years or at the point when they are 10 years younger than the age of the individual in the family when first diagnosed with the breast cancer, they should begin having clinical breast exams between two and four times a year and mammograms and MRIs annually. The optimal frequency and duration of both mammography and MRI screening in high-risk women is not known. There is some concern about long-term radiation exposure with mammography in this group; this issue needs to be further elucidated. Higher sensitivities in detecting breast cancer have been reported with MRI compared to mammogram but lower specificities. Therefore MRI is currently being used as a screening tool only in high-risk women. It is also not known whether routine MRI screening in *BRCA* mutation carriers is associated with increased survival.

The option of prophylactic mastectomy with or without reconstruction is also discussed as a potential risk-reduction strategy for *BRCA* mutation carriers. On the basis of results of retrospective and prospective studies, prophylactic mastectomy appears to decrease the risk of developing breast cancer by approximately 90% in women at high risk. Long-term prospective studies are ongoing.

In practice, more women tend to choose screening over bilateral prophylactic mastectomy. Unilateral prophylactic mastectomy is also an option for *BRCA* mutation carriers diagnosed with breast cancer. There may also be a role for chemoprevention, with tamoxifen, a selective estrogen-receptor modulator (SERM), in both premenopausal and postmenopausal *BRCA* mutation carriers. Only a few small studies have evaluated the benefit of tamoxifen as a chemopreventive agent specifically in *BRCA* mutation carriers. These studies have been inconclusive owing to limited sizes. It is believed that *BRCA2* mutation carriers may receive a greater benefit from tamoxifen than *BRCA1* mutation carriers do, as the former are more likely to develop estrogen-receptor-positive tumors, which are known to be prevented by tamoxifen. In the clinical setting, it is important to present both the risks and the benefits of tamoxifen when discussing it as an option for breast cancer risk reduction in at-risk women. As yet, there are no data on the chemopreventive benefits offered by either raloxifene (another SERM) or aromatase inhibitors (AIs) in postmenopausal *BRCA* mutation carriers.

Given the lack of efficacy of screening approaches for ovarian cancer (in particular, the shortcomings of serum CA125 levels and transvaginal ultrasound for this purpose), it is currently recommended that *BRCA* mutation carriers undergo prophylactic bilateral salpingo-oophorectomy (BSO) after they have completed childbearing and are older than 35 years of age. The fallopian tubes should be removed in addition to the ovaries because of the increased risk of fallopian tube carcinoma in *BRCA* mutation carriers. Whether the uterus should be removed, given that a small part of the fallopian tube resides there, is still controversial. Ongoing prospective studies may help answer this question. We suggest that the surgery be done by a trained gynecologist/oncologist or with one present who could carry out the surgery if required, as early-stage ovarian cancer has been detected in a small percentage of these cases. In *BRCA* mutation carriers, prophylactic BSO has been associated with as much as a 50% decrease in breast cancer in premenopausal patients.

Another controversial issue is whether premenopausal women should receive hormone replacement therapy (HRT) post oophorectomy and, if so, for how long. A number of clinics use short-term hormonal therapy only in women with severe vasomotor symptoms while others give low-dose hormone therapy until the average age of menopause. Women with a history of melanoma or fair skin should undergo annual skin examination. Men with *BRCA* mutations should have annual breast exams and prostate-specific antigen (PSA) levels measured at 40 years of age.

Li-Fraumeni Syndrome

The Li-Fraumeni syndrome is a rare autosomal dominant condition in which members of a family have early-onset breast cancer, osteosarcoma, leukemia, brain tumors, and adrenocortical malignancies. In Li-Fraumeni families, the reported incidence of early-onset breast cancer is as high as 22%, and women are often susceptible to having multiple breast cancers in addition to other cancers. In approximately 50% to 77% of cases, a mutation in the *p53* gene has been detected. The *p53* gene is located on chromosome 17 and is responsible a number of cellular functions including cell growth. Testing for a mutation in the *p53* gene can be undertaken. Breast cancer screening guidelines for *p53* mutation carriers are similar to those for *BRCA* mutation carriers. Prophylactic mastectomies are also an option. It is suggested that women in Li-Fraumeni families undergo comprehensive annual physical examinations given their risk of other cancers.

Cowden Syndrome

Cowden syndrome is another rare autosomal dominant syndrome characterized by a cluster of benign and malignant conditions: mucocutaneous lesions on the face and oral mucosa; early-onset breast cancer; benign and malignant (nonmedullary) thyroid cancer; macrocephaly; cerebellar tumors; endometrial cancer; mental retardation; hamartomas of the gastrointestinal tract; benign breast lesions;

lipomas; renal carcinoma; and uterine fibroids. Cowden syndrome is the result of a deleterious mutation in the *PTEN* (phosphatase and tensin homolog) tumor suppressor gene. Testing for mutations in the *PTEN* gene is available.

In *PTEN* mutation carriers, skin lesions often present first, at an early age. Early-onset breast cancer develops in 25% to 50% of female carriers. Women can present with bilateral breast cancer. A prior history of benign breast disease is also common.

Breast cancer screening recommendations for *PTEN* mutation carriers are the same as those for *BRCA* mutation carriers. Prophylactic mastectomy is also a risk-reduction option. In premenopausal women, endometrial biopsies are recommended every 5 years beginning between the ages of 35 and 40 years and continuing until menopause; thereafter, annual ultrasounds should be performed. In addition, an annual physical examination including urinalysis, annual thyroid ultrasound, and skin examination is recommended.

Peutz-Jeghers Syndrome

Peutz-Jeghers syndrome is a rare autosomal dominant condition characterized by freckles in infancy that may fade with age and hamartomous polyps in the gastrointestinal tract. It is also associated with a 50% risk of developing breast cancer, in addition to an increased risk of colon, pancreas, stomach, and ovarian cancers (including sex cord tumors). In 50% of cases, germline mutations in *STK11* at chromosome 19 (also known as *LKB1*) are identified. Genetic testing for this syndrome is available.

Women with Peutz-Jeghers are recommended to undergo clinical breast examinations beginning at age 20 and mammograms at age 40. Annual Pap smears and transvaginal ultrasound should begin when women are teenagers. In addition, an annual comprehensive physical examination is recommended. Men with Peutz-Jeghers syndrome should have annual testicular examinations starting at age 20.

Women Without a Family History of Breast Cancer

The following criteria are used to identify women at increased risk for breast cancer who do not have a strong family history:

▷ Women 35 years or older with a 5-year breast cancer risk of 1.66% or greater [derived using the National Cancer Institute (NCI) Breast Cancer Risk Assessment Model; www.cancer.gov/bcrisktool]

▷ Women with a prior diagnosis of lobular carcinoma in situ (LCIS) or atypical hyperplasia

▷ Women with a prior history of radiation exposure

With the exception of women who have a prior history of thoracic radiation, recommended screening strategies in women at increased risk are similar to those used for the general population. In the United States, that means clinical breast examinations every 1 to 3 years between the ages of 20 and 40, followed by the addition of mammograms every 1 to 2 years between ages 40 and 50 and annually thereafter (http://www.ahrq.gov/clinic/uspstf/uspsbrca.htm). Some physicians advise semiannual clinical breast examinations.

Women who have a history of thoracic radiation are currently recommended to undergo annual clinical breast examinations before the age of 25, and breast self-examinations with annual mammograms beginning 10 years after the completion of radiation or at age 40, whichever comes first. Although data suggest that a woman's breast cancer risk varies based on her current age, radiation dose, and use of chemotherapy, these findings have not yet been translated into clinical practice. These women need to be followed closely, which can also be done by a high-risk breast clinic. As yet, no study has evaluated the benefit of annual MRI in this population.

In addition to screening, women 35 years or older with a 5-year breast cancer risk of 1.66% or greater (derived using the NCI Breast Cancer Risk Assessment Model) or with a history of LCIS or atypical hyperplasia may benefit from chemopreventive strategies such as tamoxifen (in premenopausal and postmenopausal women) or raloxifene (in postmenopausal women). Information on these chemopreventive strategies can be found in Chapter 6. Patients can also be referred to a high-risk breast clinic for discussion of the risks and benefits of these chemopreventive strategies.

Although the focus of this chapter is women who have not been diagnosed with breast cancer, it is also appropriate to refer women diagnosed with early-onset breast cancer (younger than 50 years) without a family history and women with bilateral breast cancers, second breast cancers, and ovarian cancer to a high-risk breast clinic for risk assessment, possible genetic testing, and management recommendations.

GUIDELINES FOR ASSESSMENT AND TREATMENT OF HIGH-RISK WOMEN

Expert guidelines from groups such as the U.S. Preventive Services Task Force and the National Comprehensive Cancer Network (NCCN) have been developed to assist physicians and other health providers in identifying women who, based on family history of cancer, may have an inherited breast cancer predisposition.

The criteria listed in Table 14.1 can be used to identify woman who should be referred to a high-risk breast clinic for one or more of the hereditary breast cancer syndromes. Information on high-risk breast clinics is available on the websites of most National Cancer Institute (NCI)–designated Comprehensive Cancer Centers and many university-affiliated Breast Centers. These facilities can provide a more detailed risk assessment as well as genetic counseling and testing, breast examination and tailored screening, and risk-reduction strategies for women who are at increased risk of breast and ovarian cancers. Their staffs usually include both genetic counselors and medical oncologists/internists. When genetic testing is an option, testing of a family member affected with cancer is preferred; unaffected members would then be tested only if a mutation was found. Patients and/or family members who come to these clinics also often have the opportunity to be involved with ongoing research studies. The following websites may also be helpful in locating a high-risk breast clinic:

▷ http://www.cancer.gov/cancercenters/centerslist.html
▷ http://facingourrisk.org/finding_health_care/finding_specialists.html#clinics
▷ http://www.cancer.gov/search/results_geneticsservices.aspx

Women with a strong family history (based on the criteria outlined in Table 14.1) but no identified genetic mutation are usually managed similarly to *BRCA* mutation carriers. For the remaining women with a family history, annual clinical breast examination and mammogram screening are usually recommended to begin 10 years before the first case of breast cancer was diagnosed in the family, except if the diagnosis of breast cancer occurred while the family member was in her early twenties. MRI is currently not recommended for these women.

~ Frequently Asked Questions

1. *Once a patient is confirmed to have a deleterious BRCA1 or BRCA2 mutation, how urgent is it for her to take action if she is considering prophylactic surgery?*

   Under normal circumstances, other than increasing intensity of breast and ovarian surveillance, it is not urgent for her to take action. In fact, a woman is advised to take the time to gather opinions and discuss options with treating physicians and family members when considering all risk-reduction options. The only scenario that requires immediate action is when a patient who has breast cancer and is found to be positive for a *BRCA* mutation is considering bilateral mastectomies and reconstruction. This is because specific types of breast reconstruction, such as deep inferior epigastric perforator (DIEP) flaps, can be done only once. If this is the case, the patient should discuss this issue with her breast and plastic surgeon and be referred to a high-risk breast clinic as soon as possible, as it can take between 4 and 6 weeks to get genetic test results back pending insurance authorization.

2. *How young is it reasonable to test a patient for mutations in the BRCA1 and BRCA2 genes?*

   We usually recommend delaying testing until at least the mid-twenties, when it may affect the choice of screening strategies. In making this decision, we also take into consideration the maturity, emotional state, and wishes of the individual. We do recommend that women be seen at a high-risk breast clinic to discuss their risk and guide screening strategies, and also so that they can be informed of ongoing changes in practice as the field evolves. This can be done earlier if they are aware of their family's history of breast cancer.

At present we recommend that young women in families of known *BRCA* mutations carriers, who have not been tested themselves, perform monthly breast self-examinations from age 18 onward and undergo annual clinical breast examinations as part of their annual physical examinations. In addition, we recommend that at age 25, women in this group begin semiannual clinical breast examinations, annual mammograms, and MRIs. The starting age may be lowered if there is a very early onset of breast cancer in the family.

3. Is BRCA *genetic testing covered by insurance?*

Insurance reimbursement may vary from country to country and from place to place. In the United States, most insurance companies cover at least 80% of the cost of genetic testing. Each insurance company has its own set of criteria. If testing is believed to be clinically required, a letter of medical necessity can be sent to the insurance company.

4. Does being BRCA *positive affect a patient's health insurance or life insurance?*

In the United States, the Health Insurance Portability and Accounting Act of 1996 (HIPAA) prevents group health coverage from either excluding individuals or increasing their premiums as a result of genetic testing results. However, the same rule does not apply to individual insurance coverage. In addition, HIPAA does not prevent health insurance companies from asking about prior genetic testing.

A number of states have laws prohibiting group health plans from discriminating on the basis of genetic testing results; some states also have legislation preventing employers from discriminating on the basis of genetic testing results. There is not the same protection for disability or life insurance.

To date, it seems that genetic discrimination has not become a problem. Updated information on state-based cancer legislation can be obtained from the National Cancer Institute (www.scid-nci.net).

5. How long do BRCA *mutation carriers have to be screened?*

Testing should occur intermittently throughout the patient's life. These patients should be connected to a high-risk breast clinic so that if imaging modalities or chemoprevention approaches change, they will be aware of this fact.

FURTHER READING

Claus EB, Risch N, Thompson WD. Autosomal dominant inheritance of early-onset breast cancer: Implications for risk prediction. Cancer (Phila) 1994;73:643–651.

Fisher B, Constantino JP, Wickerham DL, et al. Tamoxifen for prevention of breast cancer: Report of the National Surgical Adjuvant Breast and Bowel Project P-1 Study. J Natl Cancer Inst (Bethesda) 1993;90:1371–1388.

Gail MH, Brinton LA, Byar DP, et al. Projecting individualized probabilities of developing breast cancer for white females who are being examined annually. J Natl Cancer Inst (Bethesda) 1989;81:1879–1886.

WEBSITES

http://facingourrisk.org/finding_health_care/finding_specialists.html#clinics
http://www.cancer.gov/search/results_geneticsservices.aspx
http://www.ahrq.gov/clinic/uspstf/uspsbrca.htm
http://www.cancer.gov/bcrisktool/
http://www.cancer.org/docroot/home/index.asp
http://www.scid-nci.net

Algorithm for the Breast Work-up

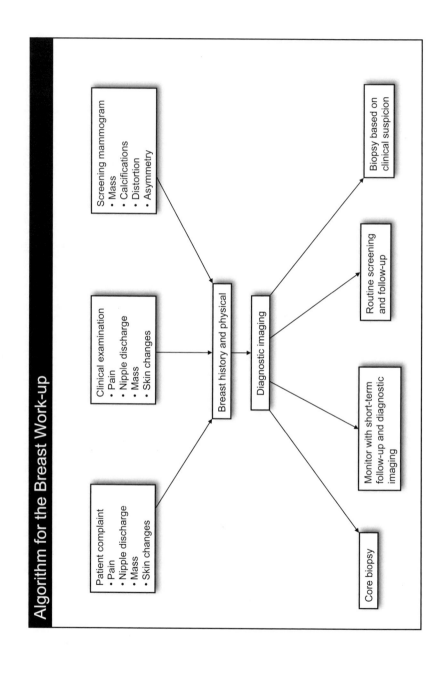

15

Benign Breast Disease

Theodore N. Tsangaris, MD

What you need to know:

Every breast problem should be approached in a consistent way. The three basic elements include history, physical examination, and diagnostic imaging.

A diagnostic mammogram should be ordered for any breast problem. This type of imaging study can and should be obtained even before the patient sees a breast surgeon. The health care provider should provide as much pertinent information as possible to aid the mammographer in the work-up.

All breast problems should be approached with a high index of suspicion and with the goal of ruling out breast cancer.

What your patient needs to know:

Most problems of the breast are benign. However, patients should be encouraged to bring any issues to the attention of their health care provider.

Breast self-examination is important in providing information about stability in a clinical finding. It may also aid the clinician and the mammographer in their work-up.

Patients should be reassured about the safety and efficacy of the core biopsy as the procedure of choice when a biopsy is necessary.

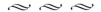

INTRODUCTION

The specific entity of benign breast disease does not exist. Rather, benign breast disease is a collection of symptoms with or without corresponding pathological findings. These symptoms are relatively unimportant as pathologic findings and are often collectively termed "fibrocystic disease."[1]

There are few effective treatments for these symptoms or pathologic findings. Surgery for this group of entities is usually not indicated but is almost always used as a diagnostic tool. Frankly, your patient will be interested in just two diagnoses of the breast when faced with a problem: cancer and "not cancer" (i.e., benign disease). Specifics and treatment of benign disease are usually not important to the patient once she hears "not cancer." Therefore it is most important for the clinician to approach all symptoms or findings in the breast with the ultimate goal of making the diagnosis of cancer or "not cancer." This chapter describes the presenting symptoms of benign breast disease and explains how to make the diagnosis of cancer or "not cancer" (benign).

GENERAL APPROACH TO THE BREAST PROBLEM

There are three ways a breast problem will present itself to the clinician. First are the symptoms or findings identified by the patient during her breast self-examination (BSE). BSE is often maligned as a screening tool, but it is still a common way that a woman identifies a breast cancer. In addition, the familiarity of the state of her breast gained from routine BSE that a woman brings to an encounter with her physician or mammographer is invaluable. Second, a problem may present itself during a clinical breast examination performed by the patient's health care provider. Third, findings may present during breast imaging, usually during a screening mammogram.

Regardless of how the issue is identified, the same principles apply. A good history is appropriate in all situations. Attention to personal breast history, family breast history, and gynecologic history are the mainstays of the pertinent information (although most women with breast cancer have no known risk factors). A skilled breast examination follows the history. Consistency in technique is more important than the mechanics of this examination. Usually the breast examination begins on the contralateral breast so that a "normal breast" can be established for direct comparison to the breast with the problem. The breast tissue technically extends from the clavicle superiorly, to just below the inframammary fold inferiorly. It extends from the lateral edge of the sternum medially and to the posterior axillary line or latissimus muscle laterally. A complete breast examination includes both breasts as well as the axillary nodes and the supraclavicular nodes.

The work-up of a breast problem always includes breast imaging. No matter what the issue under investigation, failure to obtain appropriate breast imaging would be considered a deviation from the standard of care. The primary health care provider should feel comfortable in ordering a diagnostic breast imaging study prior to the patient seeing a breast surgeon. Not only is this step appropriate, but it will facilitate the surgeon's work-up should his or her services be needed.

What constitutes appropriate imaging is another story. Therefore, a word about obtaining a diagnostic mammogram is appropriate here. Designating the study as a "diagnostic" work-up in the request is the first and most important component. Inherent in the word "diagnostic" is the implication that a qualified breast imager will oversee the process from beginning to end. Additional views, ultrasounds, or other imaging modalities such as magnetic resonance imaging (MRI) will be employed under the watchful eye of the breast imager. This also gives him or her permission to continue the work-up to its conclusion—even to perform a biopsy if needed.

Communication with a breast imager by providing the relevant history and clinical information is paramount in facilitating the correct imaging work-up. Thus an accurate description of the symptoms or findings on the requisition form is the second most important component of the imaging study. It is the responsibility of the ordering health care provider to be clear about the purpose of the study and to provide pertinent history and clinical findings to aid the breast imager in his or her task. The most common way to relay the location of a clinical finding is by using the coordinates of the clock. Of course, if all else fails, a simple crude drawing can be very effective.

The mammographer should take the work-up to its conclusion by reaching one of the following endpoints:

▷ The mammographer may perform a core biopsy.
▷ The mammographer may make a recommendation for excisional biopsy.

▷ The mammographer may recommend a follow-up study.

▷ The mammographer may recommend continued regular screening.

Mammography is not infallible; it may miss as many as 15% of cancers for reasons related to the patient's age and breast density. Therefore, it is up to the clinician to pursue clinical findings of concern, even in the face of normal imaging studies. If biopsy is recommended, then core biopsy is preferred. Suffice it to say that core biopsy is minimally invasive, is highly accurate, and preserves breast integrity should subsequent procedures be necessary. Excisional biopsy is reserved for instances in which core biopsy cannot be performed or for discordance between core biopsy results and clinical impression. The algorithm at the beginning of this chapter illustrates the basic approach to a breast problem.[2–4]

BREAST PAIN

Breast pain may be the most common complaint a woman will associate with her breast. Unfortunately, it is often the most difficult and frustrating to diagnose and treat. Although pain is not the usual presenting sign of cancer, when cancer is the cause of breast pain it is usually of an advanced stage. Reassurance is very important and often is the most important part of treatment. Breast pain should be taken seriously, however, and the usual work-up initially outlined in this chapter should ensue. First, a thorough history and clinical breast examination should be done. Often the culprit is identified in the history. Regardless of the findings, a diagnostic mammogram should be obtained.[5]

Causes of breast pain include the influence of endogenous hormones (e.g., the menstrual cycle) or exogenous hormones (oral contraceptives and hormone replacement therapy). Stimulation of the breast from well-known culprits such as caffeine, chocolate, and soft drinks is not unusual. Again, the therapeutic value of reassurance cannot be overstated. Removing the offending cause, if one is identified, can bring about relief. Heat, vitamin E, evening primrose oil, and nonsteroidal anti-inflammatory drugs (NSAIDs) are all reasonable options, but hearing the words "not cancer" may be the most effective medicine.[6]

Assuming that the clinical examination and mammographic work-up are negative, follow-up examinations and imaging are war-

TABLE 15.1 ～ Breast Pain: A Summary

Common Causes

Menstrual cycle

Exogenous hormones

Coffee or tea

Chocolate

Soft drinks or other caffeine sources

Mass or cyst

Cancer (rare, and usually advanced at the point of causing pain)

Diagnosis

History

Physical examination

Mammogram/ultrasound

Biopsy as needed

Treatment

Reassurance

Vitamin E, evening primrose oil, nonsteroidal anti-inflammatory drugs, heat

Remove offending cause

Cyst aspiration

Excision of mass

ranted at prescribed intervals or sooner should there be any change in the patient's clinical signs or symptoms. Surgery for pain of unknown etiology is strongly discouraged. Rarely does the patient obtain pain relief after the surgery, and most often the clinical picture is complicated by the addition of postsurgical pain and changes.

Table 15.1 summarizes the common causes, diagnosis, and treatment of breast pain.

NIPPLE DISCHARGE

Contrary to popular belief, nipple discharge is common and usually benign. Of all the causes of nipple discharge, breast cancer is the least common. The anxiety of patients and health care providers increases when the nature of the discharge is crystal clear and sticky, or bloody. Even in these scenarios, however, cancer is the least common cause of bloody nipple discharge; the two most common causes are duct ectasia and intraductal papilloma.

The usual thorough history and physical examination are necessary in patients who experience nipple discharge. In addition to identifying the discharge, the clinical examination should seek other findings such as a mass or a trigger point. A trigger point is the particular area of the breast that, upon palpation or manipulation, reproduces the discharge. A mass may or may not be associated with the trigger point.

A diagnostic mammogram is also a necessary component of the work-up. A duct-o-gram may be helpful in these situations.[6] The finding of an abnormality on either mammogram or ultrasound is important. For benign nipple discharge (bilateral, nonbloody, multiple ducts), reassurance is appropriate with follow-up. Concerning nipple discharge (unilateral, single duct, bloody, or any discharge associated with clinical or mammographic abnormality) should be treated with a nipple duct exploration and/or biopsy of the associated clinical or mammographic abnormality.[7]

TABLE 15.2 ～ Nipple Discharge: A Summary

Common Causes
Benign and physiologic
Duct ectasia
Intraductal papilloma
Cancer
Diagnosis
History
Clinical examination (mass, trigger point)
Mammogram/ultrasound and duct-o-gram (mass, calcifications, distortion, filling defect)
Treatment
Observation
Biopsy as needed
Nipple duct exploration

Table 15.2 summarizes the common causes, diagnosis, and treatment of nipple discharge.

NIPPLE CHANGES

Nipple changes such as itching, scaling, change in color, and erosion could be early signs of breast cancer and warrant a complete breast work-up. Nipple changes, even in the face of a normal breast examination or mammogram, may require a biopsy to diagnose occult breast cancer.

Table 15.3 summarizes the common causes, diagnosis, and treatment of nipple changes.

RASHES AND OTHER SKIN CHANGES

The breast is covered by skin and, therefore, skin rashes are possible. These conditions should not be neglected—a heightened level of suspicion should prevail. A careful history, examination, and mammogram are mandatory. After a reasonable period of observation and consultation by a dermatologist, if needed, the persistence of the problem should initiate a work-up that includes a punch biopsy.

TABLE 15.3 ∼ Nipple Changes: A Summary

Common Causes
Benign skin lesions
Trauma
Early sign of breast cancer
Diagnosis
History
Physical examination
Mammogram/ultrasound
Biopsy of nipple
Treatment
Treat the underlying cause

TABLE 15.4   ⌇   Rashes and Other Skin Changes: A Summary

Common Causes
Infection in nursing women and women of childbearing age
Generalized skin conditions
Cancer (maintain a high index of suspicion)
Diagnosis
History
Physical examination
Mammogram/ultrasound
Treatment
Short course of antibiotics or treatment by a dermatologist
Low threshold for further work-up and biopsy

It is never considered normal to have a breast infection. All breast infections have an underlying cause and should be treated with a high index of suspicion. In women of childbearing age, women who are pregnant, and nursing mothers, physiologic bases for the infection are reasonable considerations. In all other women, and particularly in peri-menopausal and postmenopausal women, a breast infection should be considered breast cancer until proven otherwise.

A short course of antibiotics is reasonable provided that a clinical examination and diagnostic mammogram are performed immediately. Inflammatory breast cancer is often confused with a benign breast in-fection. A delay in recognizing the true etiology of the skin changes caused from this virulent form of breast cancer can be catastrophic.

Dimpling, skin retraction, changes in color, and swelling should initiate the work-up cascade for the breast previously mentioned in this chapter.

Table 15.4 summarizes the common causes, diagnosis, and treat-ment of rashes and other skin changes.

BREAST MASSES

Masses may present to the patient during BSE, the physician during clinical examination, or the radiologist during breast imaging. Regardless of their presentation, all dominant or isolated breast masses require evaluation, although not all masses need to be surgically removed. Masses that are suspicious in character or that are changing require biopsy. If a mass is clinically apparent, then breast imaging is warranted; if it is mammographically detected, then a clinical examination is appropriate.

Masses may generally be divided into cystic (fluid-filled), solid (no fluid), or complex cyst (solid and cystic). A cyst should be aspirated if it is painful, enlarging, or changing, or if the diagnosis of a simple cyst is in question. Most dominant or isolated solid masses should be biopsied with either a core biopsy or fine-needle aspiration (FNA). Excisional biopsies should be reserved for equivocal core biopsies or lesions not amenable to FNA or core biopsy. Incisional biopsies should almost never be performed.

A mass may be followed clinically and/or with imaging without surgical intervention if it has benign features, has shown stability over time, or has benign cytology on FNA or core biopsy.

Table 15.5 summarizes the common causes, diagnosis, and treatment of breast masses.

TABLE 15.5 ～ Breast Rashes: A Summary

Common Causes
Benign (e.g., cysts, fibroadenomas)
Cancer

Diagnosis
History
Physical examination
Mammogram/ultrasound
Core biopsy

Treatment
Observation (for benign, stable masses)
Aspiration (for symptomatic or changing cysts)
Excisional biopsy (for symptomatic, changing masses, or core biopsy discordance)
Lumpectomy or mastectomy (for breast cancer)

CALCIFICATIONS

Calcifications of the breast are findings unique to the mammogram. Unless they are associated with other clinical findings, they are not detectable by the patient or the clinician. However, the finding of calcifications in the breast does warrant a clinical examination.

Like breast masses, calcifications have unique characteristics that can make them suspicious or benign.[8] They also have behaviors (stability or changes) that may raise or lower suspicions for breast cancer. As with masses, the preferred mode of biopsy for calcifications is core biopsy. Calcifications are biopsied using a special mammographic machine to obtain a stereotactic biopsy.[9] Excisional biopsy using wire localization is reserved for equivocal cores or calcifications not amenable to stereotactic core biopsy. In addition, calcifications may be followed without surgical intervention if they have benign features, show stability over time, or have benign histology on core biopsy.[10, 11]

Table 15.6 summarizes the common causes, diagnosis, and treatment of calcifications.

TABLE 15.6   ~   Calcifications: A Summary

Common Causes
Benign causes
Cancer
Diagnosis
History
Physical examination
Mammogram/ultrasound
Stereotactic core biopsy (for suspicious calcifications)
Excisional biopsy with wire localization (when stereotactic biopsy cannot be performed or for core biopsy discordance)
Treatment
Observation for benign calcifications
Lumpectomy or mastectomy for cancer

SPECIAL SITUATIONS

The Pregnant Female

The pregnant woman may present with all of the previously discussed problems. Unfortunately, breast cancer can also present during pregnancy and lactation. It is said that breast cancer presenting during these periods is particularly virulent, most likely because it often presents at a later stage because of a delay in diagnosis. First, the breast during pregnancy and lactation can mask or confuse the clinical picture. Second, signs and symptoms of cancer are often erroneously attributed to these physiological states. Finally, fear of adversely affecting the pregnancy may cause a delay in performing an appropriate work-up, including breast imaging and biopsy. Signs and symptoms in the breast of a pregnant or lactating woman should be as vigorously approached as when they are detected in her nonpregnant counterparts.

The Male Breast

Although such cases are rare—accounting for only 1% of all breast cancers—men do get breast cancer. It should not be considered normal for men to have any of the symptoms that have been described for women. Like women who present with complaints or abnormal clinical findings, men deserve and warrant a thorough breast work-up, including breast imaging.[12, 13]

⤳ Frequently Asked Questions

1. *I just had a screening mammogram. Why do I need a new one now?*

   Screening mammograms that are obtained more than 3 months prior to a presenting problem should be considered old. In addition, a diagnostic mammogram complements the work-up with additional views, ultrasounds, and other imaging modalities, as needed.

2. *I have no family history of breast cancer, so why do I have to be concerned about benign breast disease?*

Most women who get breast cancer have no family history or risk factors.

3. *Should I see a breast surgeon before I get any work-up or biopsy for benign breast disease?*

Obtaining a diagnostic mammographic work-up and even biopsy is appropriate and preferable, in that these measures facilitate the care of the patient should she need the services of a surgeon. They also may make the trip to the breast surgeon's office unnecessary.

4. *Isn't it better and safer to have an excisional biopsy than a core biopsy?*

Core biopsy is preferable to excisional biopsy because it is minimally invasive and maintains the integrity of the breast should further treatment be needed. Core biopsy is safe and does not cause the spread of cancer to other parts of the breast, lymph nodes, or other parts of the body.

5. *My breast infection went away after I took antibiotics, so why do I need a mammogram now?*

Infections in the breast are not normal; they should always be viewed with suspicion and their causes explained. Mammographic work-ups should always be standard after any infection.

REFERENCES

1. www.breastcancer.org/symptoms/
2. Ibitoye BO, Adetiloye VA, Aremu AA. The appearance of benign breast diseases on ultrasound. Niger J Med 2006;15(4):421–426.
3. Graf O, Helbich TH, Hopf G, et al. Probably benign breast masses at US: Is follow-up an acceptable alternative to biopsy? Radiology 2007;244(1): 87–93.
4. Kollur SM, El Hag IA. FNA of breast fibroadenoma: Observer variability and review of cytomorphology with cytohistological correlation. Cytopathology 2006;17(5):239–244.
5. www.breastcancer.org/symptoms/understand_bc/faq_symp/pain.jsp

6. Rissanen T, Reinikainen H, Apaja-Sarkkinen M. Breast sonography in localizing the cause of nipple discharge: Comparison with galactography in 52 patients. J Ultrasound Med 2007;26(8):1031–1039.
7. Richards T, Hunt A, Courtney S, Umeh H. Nipple discharge: A sign of breast cancer? Ann R Coll Surg Engl 2007;89(2):124–126.
8. Holcomb SS. Understanding mammogram microcalcifications. Nurse Pract 2007;32(6):12–15.
9. Kikuchi M, Tsunoda-Shimizu H, Kawasaki T, et al. Indications for stereotactically-guided vacuum-assisted breast biopsy for patients with category 3 microcalcifications. Breast Cancer 2007;14(3):285–291.
10. Tse GM, Tan PH, Cheung HS, et al. Intermediate to highly suspicious calcifications in breast lesions: A radio-pathology correlation. Breast Cancer Res Treat 2007: in press.
11. Liu X, Inciardi M, Bradley JP, et al. Microcalcifications of the breast: Size matters. A mammographic–histologic correlation study. Pathologica 2007;99(1):5–10.
12. Narula HS, Carolson HE. Gynecomastia. Endocrinology Metab Clinic North Am 2007:36(2):497–519.
13. Hines SL, Tan WW, Yasrebi M, et al. The role of mammography in male patients with breast symptoms. Mayo Clinic Proc 2007;82(3):297–300.

Algorithm for Clinical Trials

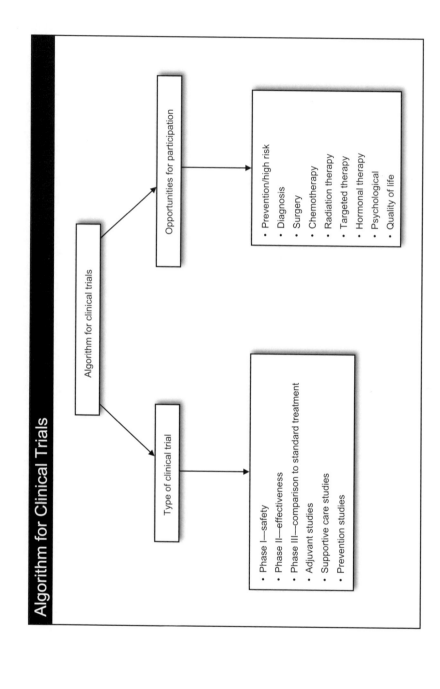

chapter

16

Talking to Patients about Participating in Clinical Trials

Lillie D. Shockney, RN, BS, MAS

What you need to know:

Approximately 85% of patients with breast cancer are unaware or unsure that they could participate in a clinical trial.

In the United States, only 3% of eligible breast cancer patients participate in a clinical trial. The most common reason that eligible patients do not enroll is because physicians fail to mention the trials to their patients.

According to research data, 93% of patients who have participated in a clinical trial found it to be a positive experience and 75% would recommend it to someone with cancer.

Several different types and levels of clinical trials exist: Phase I (tests the safety of the treatment); Phase II (determines whether the treatment actually kills cancer cells in patients); Phase III (compares standard treatments already in use with a new treatment); adjuvant studies (investigate new add-on therapies); supportive care studies (improve management of side effects); and prevention studies.

Although most laypersons associate clinical trials with chemotherapy, studies are available for participation across the continuum of care.

Please encourage your patients with breast cancer to consider participating in clinical trials. It is one way that they can receive innovative care.

What your patient needs to know:

Any current treatment women are receiving today that has been proven to be effective in the fight against breast cancer started as a clinical trial.

Patients should ask their doctors the following questions regarding participation in a study:

▷ What is the purpose of the study?

▷ How many people are included?

▷ What does the study involve?

▷ What are the risks and the benefits?

▷ How long does the study last?

▷ What type of long-term follow-up is done?

▷ Will I have any expenses?

▷ When will the results be known?

▷ Does this study specifically benefit me or is it designed to benefit the next generation of women who are diagnosed with breast cancer?

Your patient may have an opportunity to participate in clinical trials at various times during her care and treatment. Today there are clinical trials focusing on breast cancer prevention, diagnosis, surgical care, chemotherapy, radiation therapy, targeted therapy, hormonal therapy, and quality of life.

INTRODUCTION

A survey of nearly 6000 patients conducted in 2000 by Harris Interactive confirmed that approximately 85% of them were unaware or unsure that they could participate in a clinical trial. Perhaps more importantly, three out of every four patients stated that they would have been willing to enroll in such a trial had they known it was possible.[1]

Although we hope that clinical trial participation rates are better today than they were in 2000, we still have a long way to go to educate our patients about this option. In particular, participation by elderly patients and minority patients in clinical trials remains woefully low.

A panel discussion sponsored by the Susan G. Komen Foundation (www.komen.org) reported that only 3% of eligible breast cancer patients participate in clinical trials in the United States; by comparison, enrollment rates in some other countries such as Scandinavia have been as high as 70%. Reasons listed for low enrollment included failure of the physician to mention that trials existed, time requirements of physicians to explain a clinical trial, and misperceptions about the purpose of a clinical trial. There also was concern on the part of patients regarding the randomization process, even though participants are randomized to best standard therapy or to promising new innovative therapies.

The Harris Interactive survey also found that nearly one third of patients who knew about clinical trials declined to participate because they believed the new therapy would be less effective than the standard treatment; 22% feared feeling like a guinea pig. However, 93% of those patients who did participate in a clinical trial stated that their overall experience was positive, and 75% would recommend participation in a clinical trial to someone with cancer.

QUESTIONS THAT PATIENTS SHOULD ASK THEIR PHYSICIANS ABOUT CLINICAL TRIALS

It is impossible for health care providers to keep up with all of the many clinical trials that are available. It is helpful, however, if physicians and nurses interacting with the patient to mention clinical trial participation and encourage the patient to inquire about them.[2]

Following is a list of questions that patients should be encouraged to ask that may help guide them in their decision making and fact finding about clinical trials associated with their high-risk status or breast cancer diagnosis and treatment:

▷ What is the purpose of the study?
▷ How many people will be included in the study?
▷ What does the study involve?
▷ What kind of tests and treatment will I have?
▷ How are treatments given, and what side effects might I expect?

▷ What are the risks and the benefits of each protocol?

▷ How long will the study last?

▷ What type of long-term follow-up care is provided for those who participate?

▷ Will I incur any costs? Will my insurance company pay for part of them?

▷ When will the results be known?

EDUCATING PATIENTS ABOUT CLINICAL TRIALS

There are many different kinds of clinical trials. They range from studies focusing on ways to prevent, detect, diagnosis, treat, and control breast cancer to studies that address quality of life issues for patients with breast cancer. Most clinical trials are carried out in phases, where each phase is designed to learn different information and build upon previously discovered information. Patients may be eligible for studies in different phases depending on their stage of disease, therapies anticipated, and previous treatment. Patients are also monitored at specific intervals while participating in studies.

Phase I Clinical Trials

Phase I studies are used to find the best way to administer a new treatment and to determine how much of the therapy can be given safely. Only a small number of patients are asked to participate in each study. Enrollment in Phase I trials is offered to patients whose cancer cannot be helped by other known treatment modalities. Some patients have personally received benefit from participation in these studies, whereas others have experienced no benefit in fighting their cancer. Participants are, however, paving the way for the next generation, which is important.

Once the optimal dose is chosen, the drug is studied for its ability to shrink tumors in Phase II trials.

Phase II Clinical Trials

Phase II studies are designed to find out whether the treatment actually kills cancer cells in patients. A slightly larger cohort of patients is selected for this kind of trial—usually between 20 and 50. Patients whose breast cancer is no longer responding to other known treatments may be offered participation in this type of trial. Tumor shrinkage is measured, and patients are closely observed to measure the effects the treatment is having on treating their disease. If at least 20% of patients in a Phase II study respond to the treatment, the treatment is considered to be successful. Side effects are also closely monitored and carefully recorded and addressed.

Phase III Clinical Trials

Phase III studies usually compare standard treatments already in use with treatments that appeared to be effective in small-cohort Phase II trials. They require large numbers of patients to participate—usually measured in the thousands. Patients are typically randomized to one of the treatment regimens being investigated in the study. Phase III studies are seeking to show that the treatment offers benefits of longer survival, better quality of life, fewer side effects, and fewer cases of cancer recurrence.

Adjuvant Studies

Adjuvant studies are conducted to determine whether additional therapy will further improve the chance for long-term survival and reduce the risk of recurrence. Such a study progresses through Phase I, II, and III trials like other treatment studies.

Supportive Care Studies

Supportive care studies are tailored to improve ways of managing side effects caused by treatment. They also include some quality of life studies.

Prevention Studies

Prevention studies focus on patients who are at high risk for developing breast cancer or potentially having a recurrence of disease. They are commonly designed so that one group in the cohort takes a medication or some other type of therapy and the other arm of the study does not receive anything or receives a placebo. There are also some studies that focus on early detection and methods of diagnosing breast cancer sooner, even before it becomes actual cancer.

IMPROVING BREAST CANCER SURVIVAL WITH CLINICAL TRIALS

A Canadian study presented at the 4th European Breast Cancer Conference in March 2004 found that breast cancer patients who were treated according to accepted standards of care or who took part in clinical trials were 30% to 60% less likely to die from any cause during a 7-year follow-up period. This finding strongly implies that women will benefit from participation in clinical trials. Delivery of treatment in a center that treats large volumes of breast cancer patients was also associated with a higher survival rate.

The overall survival among all the women in this study at 7 years was 82%. However, when measured against women in the study who had not been treated according to accepted guidelines and who had not taken part in research, patients whose treatment followed the guidelines had 0.7 times the risk (30% less likelihood) of dying from any cause during the follow-up period, whereas women who had taken part in research had 0.4 times the risk (60% less likelihood) of dying during the follow-up period. The researchers who conducted this research studied and adjusted for key prognostic factors among these women when analyzing these data, confirming that better survival was not due to any baseline characteristics of the patients or to them being selectively chosen to participate in clinical trials.

An important message to give our patients is that a woman may derive substantial benefit from participating in clinical trials. Every successful cancer treatment being used today started as a clinical trial. Those patients who participated in these studies were the first to benefit from the new therapies. Encouraging our patients to participate can, therefore, potentially benefit our patients, but perhaps equally important to them (and, to some, even more important) may be contributing in a major way to improvements in therapy for the next generation having to deal with this disease.[3]

REFERENCES

1. Comis RL, Miller JD, Aldige CR, et al. Public attitudes toward participation in cancer clinical trials. J Clin Oncol 2003;21(5):765–766.
2. Avis NE, Smith KW, Link CL, et al. Factors associated with participation in breast cancer treatment clinical trials. J Clin Oncol 2006;24(12): 1860–1867.
3. Fukui T, Rahman M, Shimbo T, et al. Recruitment of patients for a clinical trial: Factors on the physician side and reasons on the patient side. Intern Med 2006;45(8):511–514.

Algorithm for Promoting Compliance with Breast Health Care

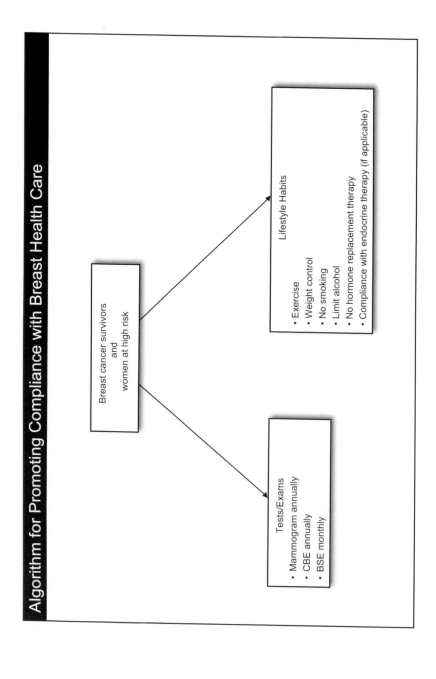

Breast cancer survivors
and
women at high risk

Tests/Exams
- Mammogram annually
- CBE annually
- BSE monthly

Lifestyle Habits
- Exercise
- Weight control
- No smoking
- Limit alcohol
- No hormone replacement therapy
- Compliance with endocrine therapy (if applicable)

chapter

17

Promoting Compliance with Breast Health Care

Lillie D. Shockney, RN, BS, MAS

What you need to know:

Even women who have had breast cancer or who are at high risk for getting breast cancer may demonstrate nonadherence to health maintenance recommendations.

Women should be encouraged and routinely reminded of the importance of consistent breast health screening, including mammography, clinical breast examination (CBE), and breast self-examination (BSE).

Selecting a breast imaging facility that provides results rapidly and offers easy access to appointments is important and helps promote compliance.

Each time you see your patient, check her chart to see when her next mammogram is due. Make sure she is comfortable performing a BSE. If she is not, arrange for someone to train her in the correct technique.

Promote healthy lifestyle habits to reduce risk. These include weight control, no smoking, and limited alcohol intake. If appropriate, refer your patient to a smoking-cessation program. Many excellent exercise programs for women are available that require a small time commitment on their part and that promote weight control and fitness. Contact the programs in your area and obtain a supply of their brochures for your office.

Hormonal therapy compliance remains an issue, despite well-documented studies demonstrating its effectiveness in the prevention of recurrence of disease in women who are breast cancer survivors as well as in the prevention of breast cancer in high-risk women. Ask your patient routinely if she is "taking her medications as prescribed" and inquire about any side effects she is experiencing that may deter her from taking the medication on a consistent basis. Talk with her oncologist, when appropriate, about whether additional measures can be taken to reduce side effects (see Chapter 9) or about switching the patient to another form of hormonal therapy if necessary.

What your patient needs to know:

Annual mammography is important for early detection of breast cancer in at-risk women. Mammography, combined with annual clinical breast examinations (and in some cases semiannual examinations for women at risk) and monthly breast self-examinations, is the key to early detection and higher survival rates for women diagnosed with breast cancer and women at high risk of developing this disease.

If the patient is not confident about how to perform a breast self-examination, arrange for a nurse practitioner to teach her the correct technique. Most Breast Centers offer this service, so a referral should be easy to make. This is a partnership you have with your patient when it comes to monitoring her breast health.

Lifestyle habits are tied to breast health. Specifically, obesity, smoking, and alcohol intake may increase the risk of getting breast cancer. Your patient needs to assume responsibility for watching her weight, avoiding smoking, and limiting alcohol consumption. If she needs help with any of these issues, she should make you aware so you can assist her. This may mean, for example, giving the patient a prescription for a smoking-cessation patch, or advising her about what type of diet to follow or which exercise programs you believe are effective.

Hormonal therapy for breast cancer prevention or reduction of risk of recurrence is to be taken daily and at the prescribed dose. If the patient has side effects that prevent her from taking her medication as prescribed, she needs to bring this matter to your attention.

INTRODUCTION

There are two groups of patients—those who have had breast cancer or who have significant risk factors for getting this disease and those who do not. The ability to instill compliance in either group at times can be more challenging than anticipated. Although it might seem logical that someone who has had breast cancer would be fearful of recurrence and want to do everything in her power to prevent such a situation, as time goes on, the foxhole religion can seemingly wear off. As a result, these survivors may join the group of women who believe they are immune to breast cancer. No matter which group your patient falls into, promoting health is something we all try to encourage.

MAMMOGRAPHY

Excuses given by patients for not wanting to get a mammogram include pain from the procedure, fear of hearing bad results, lack of health insurance coverage, lack of time, belief that mammograms cause breast cancer, lack of faith that mammograms can detect cancer early, and the anxiety of waiting to get results if an abnormality is found on the screening mammogram. In reality, studies confirm that mammography saves lives (and saves breasts). As physicians, it is part of our responsibility to spread the facts and dispel the myths about mammography, because fear of the unknown is the worst fear of all.

Following are some ways to promote compliance with screening mammography:

▷ Referring patients to a breast imaging facility that will provide results while the patient is there
▷ Ensuring easy access to appointments so patients can avoid time lost from work or other commitments
▷ Emphasizing the competence of the radiologist who is reading the images and the doctor who specializes in breast imaging modalities
▷ Identifying efficiently run facilities so that patients' time spent there is as brief as possible
▷ Educating patients about what the findings mean
▷ Offering support services to help patients cope with a diagnosis of breast cancer
▷ Providing timely feedback about the imaging results and explaining the next steps, if any are needed
▷ Making appointments available immediately for women who do have a breast abnormality or abnormal screening mammogram and need diagnostic evaluation

Ensuring that you are in the loop for getting the results promptly is also important, because your patients will rely on you for advice regarding the reported results.

Women whose health insurance does not cover screening mammograms may qualify for their state's Breast and Cervical Screening program. These programs, which are available in every state and for which eligibility is based on specific financial criteria, can offer free screening. In addition, some institutions have obtained special grants that enable them to provide free transportation and even babysitting services, with the goal of encouraging even more women to come in for annual mammography. Your local health department and American Cancer Society can provide you with information about these services. Studies have confirmed that providing a means of getting a free mammogram increases compliance.[1]

Although women continue to seek an "easier method" of breast imaging, mammography remains the gold standard for breast cancer detection today. Patients may hear stories about women whose cancer "was missed" on mammography, but it is important to reiterate to your patients at least once a year that most cancers are found at an early stage during annual mammograms.

Make reminder phone calls a day in advance to tell patients that they are expected the next day for their mammogram. Reminding them of the location of the breast imaging center and the time of their appointment helps to promote compliance and reduce no-show rates.

In addition, some physicians reward their patients for compliance with health maintenance. Something as simple as a "thank you" letter acknowledging that the patient did the right thing can be enough to promote future compliance.

CLINICAL BREAST EXAMINATION

There may be several opportunities to perform the annual clinical breast examination (CBE)—for example, at the time of the patient's annual gynecology appointment as well as when she sees her family doctor. Of course, having this opportunity requires the patient to adhere to the schedule of having an annual pelvic examination and physical examination. Take any opportunity that presents itself to perform the CBE, whether the patient is visiting her gynecologist for vaginitis or her primary care physician (PCP) for the flu. If her medical record shows that it has been 9 months or more since her last CBE, consider including it in the evaluation at that time.

BREAST SELF-EXAMINATION

When asked about breast self-examination (BSE), women often comment that they "don't know what they are supposed to be feeling for." Offering an instructional video, providing educational literature to take home including a shower card, and doing the examination with your patient will help her to understand the correct technique to use in performing this monthly exam. Although a patient may have many lumps and bumps, the goal is for her to learn what her "normal" is and to explore the breast tissue to see if there is something "new" since the last exam. Learning the geography of her breasts so she is comfortable with doing BSE is key. She should know to perform the exam a few days after her menstrual period ends or, if no longer menstruating, to select a day of the month that she will be consistently doing BSE. This will help BSE to become a habit as well as ensure that the breast tissue is at the same point in her menstrual cycle each time she does the evaluation.

It is important to reiterate that if the patient finds something during her BSE, it does not automatically mean that she has cancer. Most findings are benign. However, knowing when to call and who to call if she does find something can help ensure compliance.

Teaching young women how to do BSE beginning at age 21 can help it to become a health habit. It is a good idea to combine this education providing the facts about breast cancer and dispelling any myths that she may have heard that might instill more fear about the disease.

LIFESTYLE HABITS

There are several ways that a woman may be able to reduce her risk of getting breast cancer.

Physical Activity

Moderate activity for 30 minutes or more, 5 or more days per week, has been proven to help prevent breast cancer; exercising 3 to 5 hours per week demonstrated the greatest benefit in this regard. For prevention of breast cancer recurrence, it is recommended that patients engage in moderate activity for 30 minutes or more, 5 or more days per week; again, 3 to 5 hours of exercise per week is associated with the greatest benefit.[2]

Weight Control

Patients should consume a low-fat diet and watch their weight. Maintaining a body mass index (BMI) in the normal range for one's age group while increasing lean body mass has been found to be important in several respects:[2]

▷ Studies have shown that the risk of developing breast cancer is increased by 30% in postmenopausal women with BMIs exceeding 28 kg/m^2 compared to their counterparts with lower BMIs.[3] Premenopausal women with higher BMIs had a slightly lower risk. This difference in risk may reflect a decrease in circulating estrogens owing to the increased number of anovulatory cycles.

▷ In a prospective mortality study, the risk of recurrence of breast cancer increased with increasing BMI. There was a twofold increase in the risk of death for women with the highest BMIs (more than 40 kg/m^2) compared to those with the lowest BMIs (24.9 kg/m^2).[4]

Smoking

All patients should avoid cigarette smoke—including secondary smoke. Smoking can be one of the hardest habits to break, because it will have become a nicotine addiction for some patients. It may be helpful to discuss steps to take to achieve smoking cessation with your patients and to describe what you can offer to help wean them off cigarettes (e.g., nicotine patches). This is an opportune time to discuss how smoking affects other health issues, such as cardiac disease, hypertension, and diabetes. Clearly, avoiding smoking has many benefits.[5]

Alcohol Consumption

Most women should limit their alcohol intake to one drink per day. An estimated 2% of breast cancers are attributed to alcohol intake in the

United States; the mechanism underlying this etiology has been hypothesized to be direct DNA damage, alcohol's effects on hormone levels, or alcohol's effects on vitamin levels.[6] An adequate intake of folic acid (at least 400 μg/day) is needed to help offset the effect of moderate drinking (defined as one alcoholic beverage per day).

Ongoing Education about Breast Cancer

Patients may want to stay up-to-date on information published in credible medical journals related to discoveries associated with breast cancer risk reduction and prevention. This may be an area with which you can specifically help your patients. Consider providing consumer medical updates in your waiting room, sending periodic mailings to patients' homes, and alerting your patients to relevant educational programs offered in the community.

LINKING BREAST HEALTH WITH CHRONIC DISEASE MANAGEMENT

When your patient comes in for blood pressure checks or diabetes monitoring, take advantage of these visits and check when she last had a mammogram and CBE. Studies confirm that this kind of checking improves adherence to both breast and cervical screening.[7]

PROMOTING COMPLIANCE WITH HORMONAL THERAPY

For patients who are on long-term hormonal therapy for breast cancer prevention or to reduce their risk of breast cancer recurrence, the side effects of hormonal therapy can deter them from taking these medications as prescribed. Chapter 9 provides more information about this issue and suggests ways to increase your patients' compliance with their medication regimens.

GETTING THE WORD OUT

As a way to promote breast health habits, some Breast Centers are partnering with local colleges to hold on-campus Breastival® events, which are designed to educate college students about breast cancer and the active role they can play in reducing their risk. Some Breast Centers have partnered with local churches in an effort to reach underserved populations with their breast health message; this has also proven to be an effective way to promote compliance.

In addition, the American Cancer Society offers a free course through which laypersons can become breast health educators. This 3-hour course provides people with the tools needed to conduct a 30- or 60-minute program in their local community (for example, in parent–teacher associations and women's clubs) in which to promote screening mammography, CBE, and BSE. These programs can also provide facts and dispel myths about breast cancer and its treatment.

~ Frequently Asked Questions

1. *What are the important components of breast health assessment?*

   The most important elements are the annual clinical breast examination, annual mammogram (for women beginning at age 40), and monthly breast self-examination.

2. *Which lifestyle habits should be assessed that influence a woman's risk of getting breast cancer?*

   Risk factors for breast cancer include weight gain, smoking, excess alcohol intake, use of hormone replacement therapy (HRT), and sedentary lifestyle. Take the time to ask your patients about their exercise routine, evaluate their BMI, counsel them about not smoking (which affects the development of many other types of cancer as well as heart disease), and encourage them to limit their alcohol intake. Before prescribing HRT for any patient, you should weigh her risk of getting breast cancer against her desire to take HRT for control of menopausal symptoms.

3. *What should I tell a patient who says that she does not know what she should look for when doing a breast self-examination?*

   Put your patient in touch with a trained nurse practitioner who routinely performs clinical breast examinations for instruction in the correct technique for doing a BSE. Encourage your patient to learn the geography of her breasts and emphasize that lumps and bumps are not unusual. The important thing is to be able to identify a change in her breast geography from last month to this month. Encourage your patient to perform a BSE consistently at the same time each month.

REFERENCES

1. Phillips KA, Kerlikowske K, Baker LC, et al. Factors associated with women's adherence to mammography screening guidelines. Health Serv Res 1998;33(1):29–53.
2. Irwin ML, McTiernan A, Bernstein L, et al. Relationship of obesity and physical activity with C-peptide, leptin, and insulin-like growth factors in breast cancer survivors. Cancer Epidemiol Biomarkers Prev 2005;14(12): 2881–2888.
3. Van den Brandt PA, Spiegelman D, Yaun SS, et al. Pooled analysis of prospective cohort studies on height, weight and breast cancer risk. Am J Epidemiol 2000;152(6):514–527.
4. Calle EE, Rodriguez C, Walker-Thurmond K, Thun MJ. Overweight, obesity, and mortality from cancer in prospective studied cohort of US adults. N Engl J Med 2003;348(17):1625–1638.
5. Fentiman IS, Allen DS, Hamed H. Smoking and prognosis in women with breast cancer. Int J Clin Pract 2005;59(9):1051–1054.
6. Smoth-Warner SA, Spiegelman D, Yaun SS, et al. Alcohol and breast cancer in women: A pooled analysis of cohort studies. JAMA 1998;279(7): 535–540.
7. Coughlin SS, Uhler RJ, Hall HI, Briss PA. Nonadherence to breast and cervical cancer screening: What are the linkages to chronic disease risk? Prev Chronic Dis 2004;1(1):A04.

Resources of Benefit

The **American Cancer Society's** Breast Cancer Network
American Cancer Society, National
800-ACS-2345
http://www.cancer.org/index.html

The American Cancer Society (ACS) is a nationwide, community-based organization with chartered divisions across the country. This website is the homepage for information about clinical research trials funded by the ACS, including the Reach to Recovery program, which provides one-on-one support to newly diagnosed patients about the ACS's free programs such as Road to Recovery, I Can Cope, and Look Good, Feel Better. Also consider contacting your local ACS office for information and support.

American Society of Breast Surgeons
5950 Symphony Woods Road
Suite 212
Columbia, MD 21044
Telephone: 410-992-5470 or (toll free) 877-992-5470
Fax: 410-992-5472
General Information: contact@breastsurgeons.org
http://www.breastsurgeons.org

The American Society of Breast Surgeons was formed to encourage the study of breast surgery, to promote research and development of advanced surgical techniques, to improve standards of practice for breast surgery in the United States, and to serve as a forum for the exchange of ideas.

ASCO—American Society of Clinical Oncology
http://www.asco.org

ASCO is a nonprofit organization, founded in 1964, with overarching goals of improving cancer care and prevention and ensuring that all patients with cancer receive care of the highest quality. More than 23,000 oncology health care practitioners belong to ASCO, representing all oncology disciplines (medical, radiologic, and surgical oncology) and subspecialties.

As the world's leading professional organization representing physicians who treat people with cancer, ASCO is committed to advancing the education of oncologists and other oncology professionals, advocating for policies that provide access to high-quality cancer care, and supporting the clinical trials system and the need for increased clinical and translational research.

Cancer Information Service of the National Cancer Institute
800-4-CANCER
http://www.cancer.gov

This organization provides information about all types of cancer including excellent information about breast cancer, what it is, how it is treated, and where various treatment options are provided. You can request free information by calling the toll-free number.

CancerNet—National Cancer Institute
http://www.cancernet.nci.nih.gov
900 Rockville Pike
Building #31, HSV2580, Room 10A046
Bethesda, MD 20892
1-800-422-6237

Provides patients with information about clinical trials that may be of benefit to them.

CenterWatch Clinical Trials Listing Service
http://www.centerwatch.com
581 Boylston Street, Suite 200
Boston, MA 02116
627-247-02116

Provides clinicians and patients with information about clinical trials available in their region.

The Johns Hopkins Avon Foundation Breast Center

443-287-2778 (BRST)
410-614-2853, Lillie D. Shockney's Direct Line
Email: shockli@jhmi.edu
http://www.hopskinsbreastcenter.org

This Breast Center is one of the few comprehensive cancer centers in the country that offers state-of-the-art breast cancer diagnosis and treatment. A special feature online is Artemis, Hopkins' electronic breast cancer medical journal that you can subscribe to online for free. It is published online monthly and provides the most up-to-date information about the latest available research results and information related to the diagnosis and treatment of this disease. The website also has sections about diagnosis and treatment information, breast imaging, pathology and breast reconstruction, breast cancer patient bill of rights, and other valuable resource information.

Patients evaluated and treated at Hopkins usually meet Lillie Shockney on their first visit. She interacts with patients daily and matches the team of breast cancer survivor volunteers with women newly diagnosed based on their age, stage of disease, and anticipated treatment plan. The survivor volunteer, who has already completed the same treatment plan the new patient is about to embark on, remains connected with the patient as long as the patient desires, which is usually through and beyond the end of treatment.

The Susan G. Komen for the Cure

National Helpline 800-IM-AWARE
http://www.breastcancerinfo.com

This is a national volunteer organization seeking to eradicate breast cancer as a life-threatening disease, working through local chapters and the Race for the Cure, it sponsors events in more than 110 cities. The foundation is the largest private funder of breast cancer research in the United States. The Komen Alliance is a comprehensive program for the research, education, diagnosis, and treatment of breast disease. You will find information on their website about their mission, the accomplishments they have achieved to date, how you can participate, grants they have funded, calendar of national events, as well as other information. Komen is very big on education about the disease and on ensuring treatment for the underserved.

Mothers Supporting Daughters with Breast Cancer (MSDBC)
410-778-1982
Email: msdbc@verizon.net
http://www.mothersdaughters.org

This is a national, nonprofit organization dedicated to providing support to mothers who have daughters diagnosed with breast cancer. This organization offers a free "mother's handbook" and "daughter's companion booklet" that provides basic information about breast cancer and its treatment as well as some recommended constructive ways for mothers to provide support physically, emotionally, financially, and spiritually. The organization also "matches" mothers with mother volunteers across the country based on the daughter's (patient's) clinical picture, age at the time of diagnosis and anticipated treatment plan.

http://www.thebreastcaresite.com
This is a website sponsored by Amoena/Coloplast. It provides educational information about breast health and breast cancer, including monthly articles and an Ask the Expert section.

National Consortium of Breast Centers
P.O. Box 1334, Warsaw, IN 46581-1334
Voice: 574.267.8058
Fax: 574.267.8268
Email: wiggins@breastcare.org
http://www.breastcare.org/ or http://www.ncbcinc.org/

The National Consortium of Breast Centers' mission and purpose, according to its bylaws and articles of incorporation, is "to promote excellence in breast health care for the general public through a network of diverse professionals dedicated to the active exchange of ideas and resources, including: (1) to serve as an informational resource and to provide support services to those rendering care to people with breast diseases through educational programs, newsletters, a national directory, and patient forums; (2) to encourage professionals to concentrate and specialize in activities related to breast disease; (3) to encourage the development of programs and centers that address breast disease and promote breast health; (4) to facilitate collaborative research opportunities on issues of breast health, and; (5) to develop a set of core measures to define, improve, and sustain quality standards in comprehensive breast programs and centers."

Johns Hopkins Breast Center faculty have been directly involved in chairing the National Consortium of Breast Centers Quality Initiative, designed to facilitate the development of national quality standards for the diagnosis and treatment of breast cancer. The NCBC provides through this initiative as an opportunity to measure and assess quality of care. They also work to improve efficiency, effectiveness, and quality outcomes. PCPs and gynecologists are encouraged and welcome to attend the conferences.

National Institutes of Health
http://www.clinicaltrials.gov

Provides clinicians and patients with information pertaining to clinical trials for each type of cancer.

NCCN—National Comprehensive Cancer Network
http://www.nccn.org

The National Comprehensive Cancer Network (NCCN), a non-profit alliance of 20 of the world's leading cancer centers, is dedicated to improving the quality and effectiveness of care provided to patients with cancer. Through the leadership and expertise of clinical professionals at NCCN Member Institutions, NCCN develops resources that present valuable information to the numerous stakeholders in the health care delivery system. As the arbiter of high-quality cancer care, NCCN promotes the importance of continuous quality improvement and recognizes the significance of creating clinical practice guidelines appropriate for use by patients, clinicians, and other health care decision-makers. The primary goal of all NCCN initiatives is to improve the quality, effectiveness, and efficiency of oncology practice so patients can live better lives. NCCN offers a number of programs to give clinicians access to tools and knowledge that can help guide decision-making in the management of cancer. Johns Hopkins is a member of this alliance. At their website you will find the Breast Cancer Treatment guidelines written out for clinicians as well as a patient-friendly set to give your patients. You can also obtain hard copies of these documents from your local ACS.

People Living with Cancer

http://www.plwc.org

People Living with Cancer, the patient information website of the American Society of Clinical Oncology (ASCO), is designed to help patients and families make informed health-care decisions. The website provides information on more than 85 types of cancer, clinical trials, coping, side effects, a Find an Oncologist database, patient support organizations, and more.

Society of Surgical Oncology

http://www.surgonc.org

The Society of Surgical Oncology is a professional association for surgical oncologists and non-physician health care providers involved in oncologic patient care. On this website you will find information about our Annual Cancer Symposium, scientific journal, fellowship training programs, research grant opportunities, criteria for becoming a member, and much more. You can also obtain contact information for our 2,000-plus physician members.

The mission of the Society of Surgical Oncology is to serve its members by: (1) representing and advancing the profession of surgical oncology; (2) promoting the highest quality surgical oncology patient care outcomes, education, practice, research, ethical conduct, and advocacy; and (3) promoting public policy issues related to surgical oncology.

Y-Me National Breast Cancer Organization
800-221-2141 (24-hour national hotline)
800-221-2141 (24-hour hotline in Spanish)
Email: info@y-me.org
http://www.y-me.org

Y-Me is committed to providing information and support to anyone who has been touched by breast cancer. The services listed on their website include a national hotline for women needing emotional support, a kid's corner, referral information for approved mammography facilities near you, public education workshops where you will find a listing of upcoming events, teen programs where you can order a video specifically for teenage girls to learn about breast cancer awareness, and a resource library that provides information about treatment modalities.

Young Survival Coalition
155 6th Avenue, 10th Floor, New York, NY 10013
Tel: 212.206.6610
email: info@youngsurvival.org
http://www.youngsurvival.org

The Young Survival Coalition (YSC) is the only international, non-profit network of breast cancer survivors and supporters dedicated to the concerns and issues that are unique to young women and breast cancer. Through action, advocacy, and awareness, the YSC seeks to educate the medical, research, breast cancer, and legislative communities and to persuade them to address breast cancer in women forty and younger. The YSC also serves as a point of contact for young women living with breast cancer.

http://www.breastcancer.org
Breastcancer.org is a nonprofit organization dedicated to providing the most reliable, complete, and up-to-date information about breast cancer. Their mission is to help women and their loved ones make sense of the complex medical and personal information about breast cancer so they can make the best decisions for their lives.

WHERE CAN YOUR PATIENT GET HELP WITH FINANCIAL OR LEGAL CONCERNS?

Accompanying any serious illnesses are questions and concerns related to expenses incurred as a result of treatment, health insurance questions that can be overwhelming to try and understand or resolve alone, and sometimes even legal questions related to employment or financial matters. The following is a list of national resources to aid you in addressing these types of concerns.

Cancer Care, Inc.
212-302-2400
800-813-HOPE
Email: info@cancercare.org
http://www.cancercare.org

Cancer Care is a national, nonprofit organization that provides free, professional assistance to people with any type of cancer and to their families. This organization offers education, one-on-one counseling, financial assistance for non-medical expenses, and referrals to community services.

Credit Counseling Centers of America (CCC America)
800-493-2222
http://www.cccamerica.org

CCC America is a nonprofit organization that provides a wide array of consumer and creditor services for individuals and families experiencing financial distress.

Health Insurance Association of America
202-824-1600
800-879-4422
http://www.hiaa.org

Health Insurance Association of America is a lobbyist group for insurance companies. They can help answer questions regarding health insurance coverage.

Hill-Burton Free Care Program
800-638-0742
In MD call 800-492-0359
http://www.hrsa.dhhs.gov/osp/dfcr/

This is a national government agency that provides referrals for free medical care at participating medical facilities and most hospitals, and helps low-income individuals pay their medical bills.

National Association of Hospital Hospitality Houses, Inc.
PO Box 18087
Asheville, NC 22814-0087
828-253-1188
800-542-9730
Email: helpinghomes@nahhh.org
http://www.nahhh.org

National Association of Hospital Hospitality Houses, Inc. is a service organization of hospital hospitality houses (HHH). Member houses provide a variety of services—primarily no-cost or low-cost housing for families and patients requiring hospital treatment or care away from their homes. At present, there are approximately 150 HHH-type facilities in the United States and Canada.

National Coalition for Cancer Survivorship (NCCS)
301-650-8868
877-NCCS-YES
Email: info@ccansearch.org
http://www.cansearch.org

This network of independent groups and individuals provides information and resources about cancer support, advocacy, and quality-of-life issues as well as helping cancer patients deal with insurance or job discrimination and other related legal matters.

Patient Advocate Foundation
757-873-6668
800-532-5274
Email: patient@pinn.net
http://www.patientadvocate.org

This organization provides educational information about managed care/insurance issues and legal counseling on debt intervention, job discrimination issues, and denials of insurance coverage.

Social Security Administration (SSA)
Office of Public Inquiries
800-772-1213
http://www.ssa.gov

The SSA is the US government agency that runs the Social Security Program. It can provide information about retirement and disability benefits, supplemental security income (SSI), and Medicare.

Together Rx Access™
http://www.togetherrxaccess.com/

With the free Together Rx Access™ Card most cardholders save 25% to 40% on more than 275 brand-name prescription drugs and other prescription products, as well as on a wide range of generic drugs. There is a list of eligible drugs on the website, which can be accessed from the homepage. The Together Rx Access™ Card is sponsored by some of the world's largest pharmaceutical companies, helping more people take care of their health. Those companies are Abbott Laboratories; AstraZeneca; Bristol-Myers Squibb Company; GlaxoSmithKline; Janssen Pharmaceutica Products, L.P.; LifeScan, a Johnson & Johnson Company; Novartis Pharmaceuticals Corporation; Ortho-McNeil Pharmaceutical, Inc.; Pfizer Inc, Sanofi-Aventis; Takeda Pharmaceuticals North America, Inc.; and TAP Pharmaceutical Products, Inc.

Index

page numbers followed by *f* denote figures; those followed by *t* denote tables